FIT FEMME AFTER 50

A BUSY WOMAN'S GUIDE TO A STRONG, ATTRACTIVE, PAIN-FREE BODY

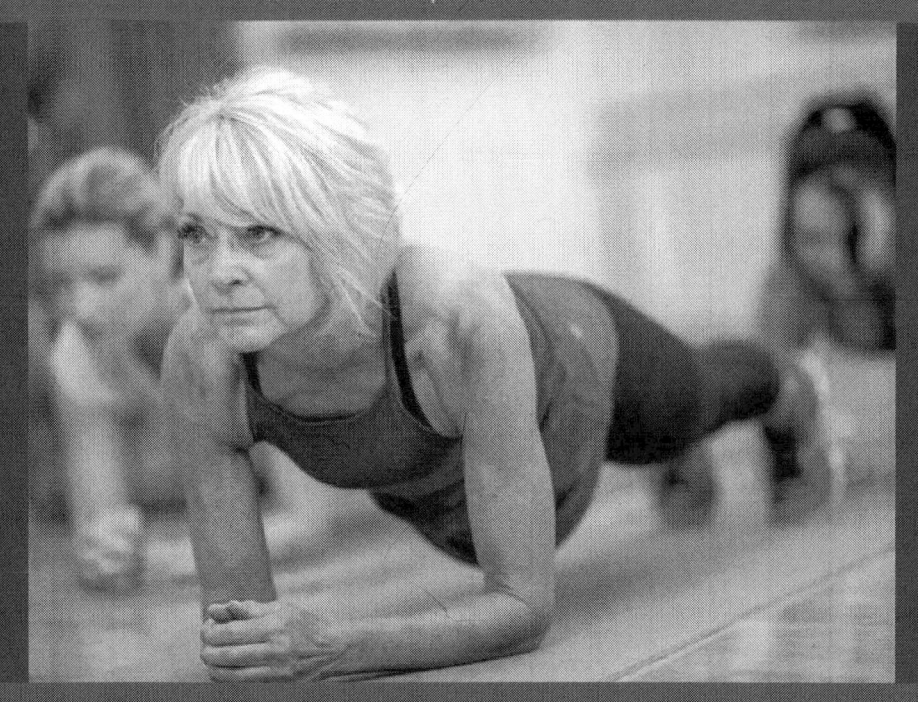

DOUG SETTER

FIT FEMME AFTER 50. Copyright © 2020 by Doug Setter.

All rights reserved. Printed in the United States of America. No part of this book may be used or reproduced in any manner without written permission except in the case of quotations embodied in articles and reviews.

ISBN: B08W7SMPCD

ACKNOWLEDGEMENTS

Writing a book is the easy part. It is the refining and promotional parts that I could not do alone. Fortunately for me, I was graced with the help of people both willing and skilled in the areas I faltered.

First, this project would not have made it at the speed it was accomplished without the guidance of Kimberly Day and her Write and Grow Rich course. I am also grateful to my costudents for their input.

Then there was the patience, humor and instruction from Barb Herda -exercise-to-music and resistance training-, Tricia Keith -Ashtanga yoga-, Tricia Dong -kettlebells-, Tina Bui -dancing- and Monique Lavoie -Pilates-. Most of all, I thank my girlfriend, Patricia Chang, for her support and putting up with me in general.

There would have been very little human interest without the personal stories of Ruby Carey, Monika Kriedmann-Bleckenwegner, Jennifer Kurtz, Iris Davis, Carol Wray, Susan Hyrnchuk and Colleen Wynia. You iron ladies rock.

Thank you to Kenric Yuen for coming up with the book title: Fit Femme After 50. Well done.

Special thanks to Dwaipayan Mani for his book cover art and patience. After nearly a dozen edits, we finally got it right -for now-.

CONTENTS

CHAPTER 01: Fit femme after 50 mindset: reprogramming to win — 6
    Programming success behavior — 8
    Positive reinforcement — 8
    Premack principle — 10
    Change your environment — 11
    The five-minute rule — 12
    Jennifer's story — 13

CHAPTER 02: Happy hormones — 15

CHAPTER 03: Posture, power and -less- pain — 21
    Posture exercises — 24
    Susan's story — 39

CHAPTER 04: Take a breath — 40
    The big stamina breathing secret — 41
    Abdominal breathing, complete breathing, and the cleansing breath — 42
    Colleen's story — 44

CHAPTER 05: Eating, energy and entertainment — 47
    The foods that support you — 50
    What to avoid — 52

CHAPTER 06: Functionally fit — 57
    Training — 58
    Lightweight resistance training exercises — 61
    Body-weight exercises -bwes — 71
    Iris davis: 76-year-old bodybuilding champion — 78

CHAPTER 07: Pain, who needs it?   **80**
    Muscle imbalance   82
    Inflammation   83
    Herbs and supplements for joint pain   86

CHAPTER 08: Nature's loan shark   **88**
    How to get a good night's sleep   90

CHAPTER 09: Brain boost   **91**
    You are smarter than you think   92
    Practical ways to improve your mind   93

CHAPTER 10: Detoxing the body, mind and spirit   **96**
    Cleansing the body   98
    Cleansing the mind   99
    Cleansing the spirit   100
    The 24-hour body-mind-spirit detox   100

CHAPTER 11: Beating the blues   **102**
    Exercise   103
    Nutrition   104
    Environment   107
    Ruby's story   107

CHAPTER 12: Roadblocks, detours and open highways   **109**

Resources   **112**

CHAPTER 01

FIT FEMME AFTER 50 MINDSET REPROGRAMMING TO WIN

FIT FEMME AFTER 50 MINDSET REPROGRAMMING TO WIN

Dressed in a bikini, the woman walks up to the chin-up bar and performs five pull-ups, then some hanging leg raises. A few days later, Iris Davis steps onto the stage of a body building competition. She takes first place. Ms. Davis is seventy-six years old.

Monika Kriedmann-Bleckenwegner has a tooth pulled the day before the Austria Iron Man competition. The next day, the fifty-plus-year-old insurance and wealth protection specialist swims 2.4 miles -3.86 km-, then bicycles 112 miles -180.25 km- and finishes off the race with a full 26.2 mile -42.2 km- marathon. After the race, the pretty blonde enjoys local beer and Austrian food.

In her sixties, Carol Wray instructs yoga to hundreds of people including athletes, firefighters and martial artists. A university graduate and former grocery store worker, the mother of two travels around the world, kayaks, canoes, and hikes regularly. -Both of her daughters are athletes, with one recently setting a world record in cycling.- A strict vegetarian, Carol still enjoys beer and good wine.

Each of these female powerhouses all have different training programs, diets, lifestyles and motivations for staying strong and healthy. Yet they all possess a winning mindset toward good health, fitness and life, for that matter. Unlike most of the population, these ladies love exercise and leading active lives.

What's more, none of them are super rich celebrities who can afford the best spas, personal trainers, rejuvenation methods or plastic surgeons. In fact, I found just the opposite. Many of these healthy, over-fifty-year-olds have experienced setbacks and personal tragedies.

Not to worry if you are one of those souls who sees exercise as embarrassing or a bitter medicine. This chapter is dedicated to reprogramming your mind to support healthy habits so that thinking about good nutrition, sleep, exercise, etc. becomes part of your lifestyle.

And the excuse of being past the half-century mark does not work. If a C+ average high school student can attend university at age sixty or a former cancer patient and auto crash survivor can win a fitness contest at age fifty, then you can still improve your strength and health. And why not? You have too many years of good living to enjoy.

So for the next few pages, let's just put the blame game on hold. You know, all of the degrading things that school kids, teachers, parents and adults said and did that made you feel that you were not good enough. In fact, all of the high performers whom I interviewed have had setbacks and tragedies in their lives. They do not see themselves as helpless products of their past.

Yesterday is gone.

PROGRAMMING SUCCESS BEHAVIOR

It is our behavior that will often determine our successes and failures in our future. For this reason, healthy thoughts and actions will most likely result in healthy outcomes in your life.

The trick is to develop these habits on autopilot so you do not need willpower to force yourself to do them. That way, you don't even have to think about exercising, eating healthy, sleeping regularly, working, studying and socializing.

Here is where the science of behaviorism can help us reprogram our minds away from those deep-seated destructive habits and develop positive, healthy habits. Trust me on this: Sometimes it can feel like a daily war with yourself. But let's work with what we have and do the best that we can

POSITIVE REINFORCEMENT

This is most effective when you give yourself SMALL, IMMEDIATE rewards for doing something positive. This might mean eating an apple or a good sit-down meal, a telephone call with a friend, reading a magazine or watching a favorite television show AFTER you have exercised or completed a task.

In my university years, I applied positive reinforcement when my studying and writing was sadly lacking. I had to build a reward system to make sure that I read the material and studied the textbook chapters.

For every four pages or whole chapter that I read of a textbook, I allowed myself to read at least four pages of fiction. So when I got on the bus to go to university and come home, I read four pages from a textbook, then four pages of fiction. I did this twice a day, five times a week for four weeks and noticed that my biology marks went from Ds to Bs.

Reading four pages, twice a day, five days a week for four weeks. That meant reading at least 160 pages a month. It is just like walking an extra distance each day. The small efforts add up.

If your new behavior is going to be exercising, then you can try a positive reinforcement program like rewarding yourself with a tea, talking to a friend, a favorite television show or any activity you enjoy for every fifteen minutes of walking, running or other exercise.

Say you want to accomplish fifty abdominal crunches per day. Here's what that might look like while taking advantage of positive reinforcement: In the morning you do an easy two sets of ten, then clean up and reward yourself with breakfast. When you get home or to the gym, you again perform another two sets of ten in front of the television. Your reward can be supper. Just before bedtime, you do another set of ten. Then reward yourself with some reading.

After a couple of weeks, the fifty crunches can easily turn into a more advanced abdominal routine that you only need to do twice a week.

Small efforts followed by small rewards.

Many of the women in my cardio kickboxing class used to work out before one of their favorite television shows -e.g. ER, Survivor, etc.-. After exercising, they often sped home to clean up, have supper and be rewarded with their favorite entertainment.

See that? They quickly rewarded themselves, during and immediately after their exercise class. So, their evening was full of positive reinforcements:

- When they arrived at the cardio kickboxing class, they may have made some friends. Reward #1.
- Next, they had a -hopefully- fun experience training with what I called the hard-hitting, sweat-pouring, aggression-releasing, kickboxer-inside- of-us-all workout. Reward #2.
- Then they -hopefully- felt elevated and stress free after the workout. Reward #3.
- Finally, after they left, they might have socialized with friends or went home to a refreshing shower, hot meal and fun television show. Rewards #4, #5 & #6.

Now, the long-term benefits of improved coordination, strength, endurance and weight loss could be motivating factors. But those are delayed reinforcements. Though the rewards are bigger and long lasting, they are too separated from the exercise to build a strong link to your behavior.

With all of the good, positive feelings associated with the exercise class, it was easy to keep showing up. The positive feelings often outweighed the fatigue, the night before, the bad sleep, the bad day at work, or the frustration with a spouse or customer.

What NOT to do: This positive reinforcement method will seldom work if you offer yourself LARGE REWARDS after LONG DELAYS. The prime example being the person who promises themselves a Victoria Secret outfit or trip to Maui if they can lose twenty pounds before the summertime. This type of conditioning is flawed, as your brain does not see the immediate reward with exercising. Your brain will tend to separate the two activities.

To strengthen this kind of delayed reinforcement, you should do something during or immediately following your exercise routine. This is as simple as making a chart or a calendar and recording your progress. Each check mark and each act of writing down what you did will help you focus on that goal. Otherwise, the demons of distraction can cloud your mind and lead you elsewhere.

So, here is your PLAN to reprogram your exercise habits.

1. Select an exercise routine, such as walking ten blocks, running two miles, fifty crunches, yoga class, or thirty minutes of weightlifting two or three times a week. Keep it simple if you are just starting out.
2. Choose a small, immediate reward, such as meeting a friend, gourmet tea, your favorite television show, a healthy snack, reading a novel, combing your hair, or even talking on the telephone.
3. Mark down on your calendar -keep track- whenever you perform your exercises.

PREMACK PRINCIPLE

The Premack principle is linking a probable activity with a less probable activity. A good example of this doing is something enjoyable, such as listening to music or socializing, while running, exercising, or working. Listening to music -probable- begins to link with exercising -less probable-.

Another example is the person who often needs to smoke cigarettes whenever they talk on the telephone. The two activities become linked together.

I once asked a sixty-seven-year-old owner of a moving company and Arnis -stick-fighting- instructor how he built his muscles. -This guy Dante was ripped!- He explained that he ate well and exercised while watching television. So, he often felt the urge to exercise when watching television. "One time," he said, "I did a thousand leg raises."

This Premack principle can be used throughout the day as well. Whenever you get to your car, desk, worksite, classroom, etc., you can tell yourself that you are going to have a great day. After a while, you will automatically think positive thoughts when you arrive at these places.

CHANGE YOUR ENVIRONMENT

"You are a product of your environment. So, choose the environment that will best develop you toward your objective." - W. Clement Stone

Ever notice how you pick up habits when working at different jobs, living in foreign countries, or hanging around certain people and places? It might be why some people become more successful when they move to a new location or job. This is why your environment can be so important for achieving a healthy lifestyle.

There are four basic environment changes that you can make to improve your exercise -studying, working, whatever- behavior:

- Location
- Position within the location
- Other people
- Time

D. Location. Sometimes in the military, I was forced to do what we called CB -Confined to Barracks- workouts. That is, I did squats, sit-ups and push-ups in the space by my bunk. It was hard to focus and stay motivated whereas working out at a gym, dojo or studio was far easier and more energizing.

E. Therefore, find a location where you like exercising. It can be a park, gym, beach or a special room with art and music that you like. The positive environment will often trigger your exercise behavior.

F. Position. Sometimes even a good location can have a better location within it. For instance, I prefer to work out around the free weights or the empty exercise room rather than be near the machines and treadmills where the fashion show and socializers are.

G. Other people. It is more energizing to train around energized people than slackers. I prefer to train around younger, motivated people or athletes. I avoid the moaners and procrastinators. As multimillionaire Dan Pena insists, "Show me your friends and I'll show you your future."

H. Time. Find a consistent time to exercise -or whatever habit you're encouraging-. This way, like with meals, work and bedtime, your mind will start preparing for that specific time to exercise. Personally, I like to spend a few minutes in the morning to walk, exercise or meditate. It starts the day off right and has become my habit. If your best time is 6 p.m. after work, then so be it. Again, strive to be consistent.

THE FIVE-MINUTE RULE

Are you still stuck in procrastination?

I often use the five-minute rule when it comes to housecleaning, writing an article, studying from a textbook or getting in that late-night workout.

Simply tell yourself that you can do the chore for only five minutes. Anyone can do something unpleasant like scrub a toilet, vacuum a rug, read a textbook or talk to an irate customer on the telephone for five short minutes. When you do this, you will often find that you can keep going for a longer time.

I often use the five-minute rule if I go to a running track on a cold, damp day and am feeling all of the motivation of a three-toed sloth. I know that I can at least run for five minutes. So I start jogging, cursing the weather and my stiff muscles. Then the magic happens. After the first two or three minutes, I start to feel better -and think "What the heck?"- and then end up running and training for thirty minutes or more. I find the same thing with housecleaning or studying. Once engaged for five minutes, the momentum carries me along.

It is the start that stops most people. So, use the five-minute rule whenever you can.

JENNIFER'S STORY

Jennifer never worked in the fitness industry. Her passion was interior design, specializing in restaurants. The bulk of her work was sedentary and put her close to food for most of her working hours. When she was in her thirties, she belonged to the local YWCA but was not really committed. By the time she was forty, she was overweight and wearing a size 12.

Her lifestyle-shifting pivot point came when she was forty-two and on a business trip. After a random meeting with a very fit man who trained with kettlebells, Jennifer changed her fitness mindset.

"I did the Insanity DVD every day and dropped forty pounds," she explained. "I went from a size 12 to a 4, then sometimes 2. From there, my size and weight went up and down. But never to the extreme.

"I love food. Since I design restaurants, dining on good food is part of my entertainment, and I can get really obsessive over food if I want to.

"I have a clean diet. I don't buy premade stuff. I drink wine once or twice a week. I once went through a phase of very clean eating and losing weight. This was when I physically could not drink alcohol at all. With the COVID restrictions, I really look forward to dinner at the end of the day. You might say that food can be my reward.

"I used to follow the New Year's resolution crowd until one year, I just decided to go easier on myself. I just do something physical every day. From 2012 to 2019, I completed over a thousand barre fitness classes, and in 2019 I was mostly training in Pilates. But I found myself in a rut and now work with a trainer twice a week.

"Five to seven years ago, my goal was to weigh 119 pounds. Now, I no longer get twitchy over my scale -which no longer works-. I train for strength now. My typical targets are to do a pull-up and press into a handstand. With my trainer, I alternate with squats and deadlifts during the week. I got my pistol squat a few weeks ago and can now deadlift 120 pounds, three reps times three sets. I also hired a swimming instructor to help work on my endurance. I love it!"

In January 2021, Jennifer will be fifty-one years old. She still runs her own design business: www.kurtzdesign.ca

SUMMARY

- Plenty of people are self-programmed to live strong, healthy lives.
- Program yourself to exercise by using one or a combination of the following:
  - Positive Reinforcement
  - Premack Principle
  - Controlling Your Environment
  - The Five-Minute Rule

START NOW!

Your contract:

I am going to exercise for minimum_____minutes by doing_____. I will do this_____times a week at this time:_____.
I will reward myself with_____,_____&
_____.

Signed _____   Date _____
Witness _____   Date _____

KEEP GOING!

CHAPTER 02

HAPPY HORMONES

HAPPY HORMONES

Hormones are always joked about and seldom taken seriously. That is, until health fails, moods swing and energy fades. Our body's messengers have lots to say about how we feel and act, so we should pay attention to them.

Wouldn't it be great to have both the reasoning of a mature mind and the youthful energy of a strong hormonal system? Following are just a few of the hormones that you should be looking after.

HUMAN GROWTH HORMONE HGH

Now, before anyone runs away at the sound of the words "growth" and "hormone," let me just say that it has many important functions in the human body. It can

- Repair your body quickly
- Fight infection
- Build muscle
- Burn fat

I have used nutrition supplements that naturally release HGH with good results. When I was taking about 500-1,000 mg -1 gram- of the amino acid L-arginine per day, my strength increased, but I became much leaner. Also, any injury such as a cut would heal very quickly.

I also used arginine just before dental surgery. The oral bleeding stopped within an hour of the operation, and I did not need any of the prescribed painkillers. Months later, when I had stopped taking the arginine and had a similar operation, I was bleeding for several hours afterward. And I ended up using all of the prescribed painkillers from both operations.

Your body's levels of human growth hormone are activated by

- Fasting
- Sleep
- Peak exertion exercise, such as weightlifting, isometrics and body-weight exercises
- Supplements such as arginine and ornithine

ADRENALINE

I am sure that you have had those times in your youth where a good hit of adrenaline made you faster and stronger than you thought possible. It even got you out of some bad situations.

These good adrenaline rushes can be healthy and even addictive. When the body is under enjoyable high-adrenaline stress, it rebuilds itself faster than with the milder, much safer, low-stress exercises like jogging. This is to say, alpine skiing has certain body and mind benefits that cross-country skiing lacks.

Adrenaline can also protect you in times of stress. When you are pumped full of adrenaline, you can often work harder and take more pain than you thought possible.

The problem is when adrenaline gets stuck "on." Then, it keeps your body in a constant state of high excitement, even though the danger has passed. This can lead to a host of symptoms such as teeth grinding, fatigue, insomnia, PMS, lower back pain, frequent accidents, and inability to concentrate. Living in a constant state of stress can destroy your health.

To tame adrenaline, we need to give it a break and feed the adrenal glands. After all, your adrenal glands are designed to protect you and take you into old age.

Take a look at the following steps to reduce adrenal exhaustion:

- Reduce coffee, nicotine, alcohol and other stimulants.
- Exercise and allow for recovery.
- Get quality sleep.
- Take multi-B and calcium-magnesium -2:1- supplements to replace depleted nutrients.

ESTROGEN

Estrogen -female hormones- regulates the menstrual cycle and, reportedly, the female biological love of chocolate.[ii] Low levels of this hormone can affect your mood, libido and generally your health. Maintaining estrogen can be done mostly through staying healthy through the exercise and nutritional recommendations.

To promote the production of estrogen

- Eat soybeans, flaxseed, wheat germ and sesame seeds.
- Take 400-800 IU of vitamin E.

- Take the herb dong quai.
- Exercise.

INSULIN

Insulin's job is to stabilize your blood sugar. This is important because as little as half a teaspoon too much or too little of sugar in your bloodstream can put you into a state of shock or a coma. The balance is that delicate. When excess sugar hits the bloodstream, causing blood sugar to spike, the body releases insulin to stabilize blood sugar. This overcompensation of insulin causes a drop in blood sugar, which makes most people feel tired. So, rather than wait for the fatigue to pass, the average person seeks out another hit of sugar to maintain alertness. And the cycle continues.

You can see the effects of candy on children. They often undergo mood changes, aggression and hyperactivity, followed by a state of grogginess.

This is why I am a big believer in a low-glycemic diet. This is mostly high protein and complex carbohydrates. -See the menus in Resources.- Even if you must have that high-sugar item, like a pastry, ensure that you eat some kind of protein first to slow down the sugar spike. This can be something as simple as a piece of cheese, hard-boiled egg or almond butter on crackers.

You can support your insulin in these ways:

- Eat high-protein and complex-carbohydrate meals -see the low-glycemic foods-.
- Exercise regularly.
- Get regular sleep.
- Some scientific papers report that 500-1,000 mcg of chromium picolinate or chromium polynicotinate can stabilize blood sugar and reduce the incidence of type 2 diabetes. It is generally harmless and worth taking note of.

CORTISOL

Cortisol protects the body during times of stress and injury. It raises blood sugar levels, enhances your brain's use of glucose, reduces inflammation -hence cortisone shots from the doctor- and increases your body's ability to repair itself. It also decreases nonessential body functions -like digestion- during times of stress.

Like other stress hormones -e.g. adrenaline-, too much cortisol can deplete your muscles and bones of nutrients, cause weight loss/gain, and disrupt your body's ability to repair itself. If you have suffered from trauma, you may find that your cortisol levels are excessively high. Excess cortisol can lead to[iii]

- High blood pressure
- Flushed face
- Weight gain in face and abdomen
- Muscle weakness
- Increased thirst
- Moodiness and irritability
- Frequent urination -late-night washroom visits-

To lower your cortisol levels, take the following steps:

- Get good quality sleep.
- Take fish oils.
- Take magnesium supplements -minimum 400 mg per day-.
- Learn to relax through hobbies, socializing and meditation.
- Exercise, but do not overdo it.
- If you like dancing, consider ballroom or Latin dancing instead of nightclub dancing.

Here is an interesting study regarding dancing: Psychology professors Cynthia Ouiroga Murcia, PhD, and Stephan Bongard from the Goethe University Frankfurt and musicology professor Gunter Kreutz from the Carl von Ossietzky University conducted a study on the effects of tango dancing on the dancer's stress hormonal levels.

What they found was that regular dancing with a partner and music lowered the cortisol levels in both male and female dancers. Dancing alone or without music was significantly less beneficial than dancing with a partner and with music. Nightclub dancers burned more calories and had higher cortisol levels.

Males who danced registered higher testosterone levels than males who passively listened to music. So, men also benefit from dancing.

GREHLIN

Grehlin induces hunger when your stomach is empty. But the more you eat, the more you produce grehlin. For most people, regular meals work better than eating throughout the day. Lack of sleep will also produce more grehlin and cortisol and increase a craving for sugary snacks. Hence, many sleep-starved late-shift workers tend to be overweight.

To prevent too much grehlin

- Get enough sleep.
- Avoid eating too much sugar.
- Do not eat too often.
- Eat more protein.
- Practice intermittent fasting.

Intermittent fasting is just skipping a meal or two or giving yourself a day for resting your digestive system. It's a good method for resetting your hormonal system. It is not recommended if you are working hard, especially in cold weather.

THYROID HORMONES: Thyroxine -T4- and Triiodothyronine -T3-

The thyroid is the body's thermostat for converting oxygen and calories into energy. People with hypothyroidism -low thyroid- problems tend to have low energy, depression, weight gain and tobacco and alcohol cravings. It is the body's supply of iodine that works with the amino acid tyrosine -used in the Red Bull©drink- to form T3 and T4. Reportedly, consuming extra iodine from seafood, iodized salt or supplements can relieve hypothyroidism symptoms.

A hyperactive thyroid is a different situation and should require the treatment of a physician.

For healthy thyroid hormones, consume iodine-rich foods and supplements. Also avoid iodine-blocking foods like Brussels sprouts, cauliflower, turnips, cabbage, kale, broccoli, and bok choy.

CHAPTER 03

POSTURE, POWER AND -LESS- PAIN

POSTURE, POWER AND -LESS- PAIN

I want to get old gracefully. I want to have good posture. I want to be healthy and be a good example to my children." - Sting

"Good posture and an attitude let you get away with anything." - Lorna Landvik, author and comedian

"Because of poor posture, practically 95% of our population suffers from varying degrees of spinal curvature. Not to mention more serious ailments." - Joseph H. Pilates, creator of the Pilates system

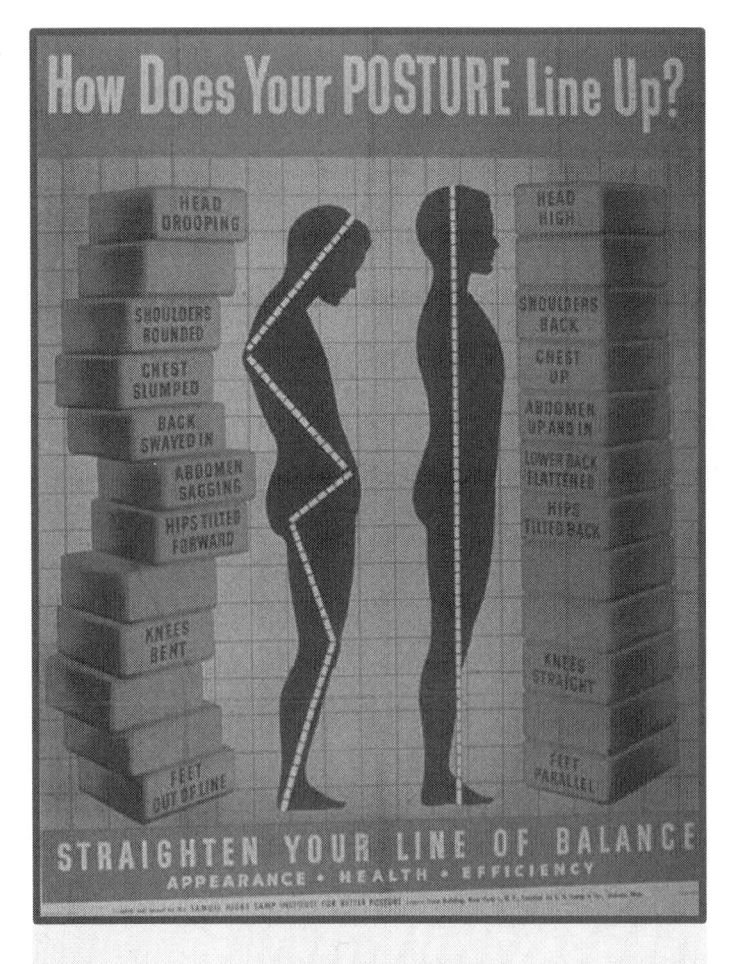

Poster from Office of Emergency Management 1941 to 1945

If you look long enough at the postures of people around you, you will start to notice that people with good posture are healthier and more confident than most of the population. Even on television, you will notice that most of the news announcers, actors, reporters and even politicians tend to have good posture. Good posture not only projects confidence-it develops strength and health.

The army and practicing martial arts drilled a straight posture into me. I soon noticed how much more weight I could lift and carry when my posture improved.

After my fortieth birthday, I discovered Pilates and different forms of power yoga, which further improved my posture AND reduced my shoulder, back, hip and knee pain. It appeared that much of my chronic pain was more from muscle imbalance than injuries. Therefore, when my body became more aligned, I could train longer without pain.

A strong posture also assists in proper digestion. I never could understand how some people can function while slumped over their desks, leaning on the bar, or slouched in front of the television set for hours and hours. These warped postures not only can lead to pain and fatigue, but they also inhibit proper digestion and breathing.

Think about that. Poor digestion and shallow breathing can cause fewer nutrients and less oxygen getting to your brain and body, and waste products not being removed. Do you think that this oxygen and nutrient starvation might affect your health and mood? Just how long can you fake it with coffee and stimulants?

Here is where the science of good body alignment will save you pain and fatigue, and maybe even get you more dance partners.

The following exercises are designed to stretch and strengthen weak posture areas such as the upper and lower back, hip flexors, abdominals, and hamstrings. Like any exercise, first consult your health practitioner and start gradually. These exercises have worked for dozens of people, including yours truly, time and again. Often an improvement can be felt after only one session.

POSTURE EXERCISES

CAT STRETCH

This is a great exercise to stretch the spine and strengthen the abdominal muscles. It is very useful for heavier people who feel pressure on their lungs when they try to perform sit-ups or crunches while lying on their backs. Most gyms do not recognize this and expect obese members to do crunches and sit-ups like an average person.

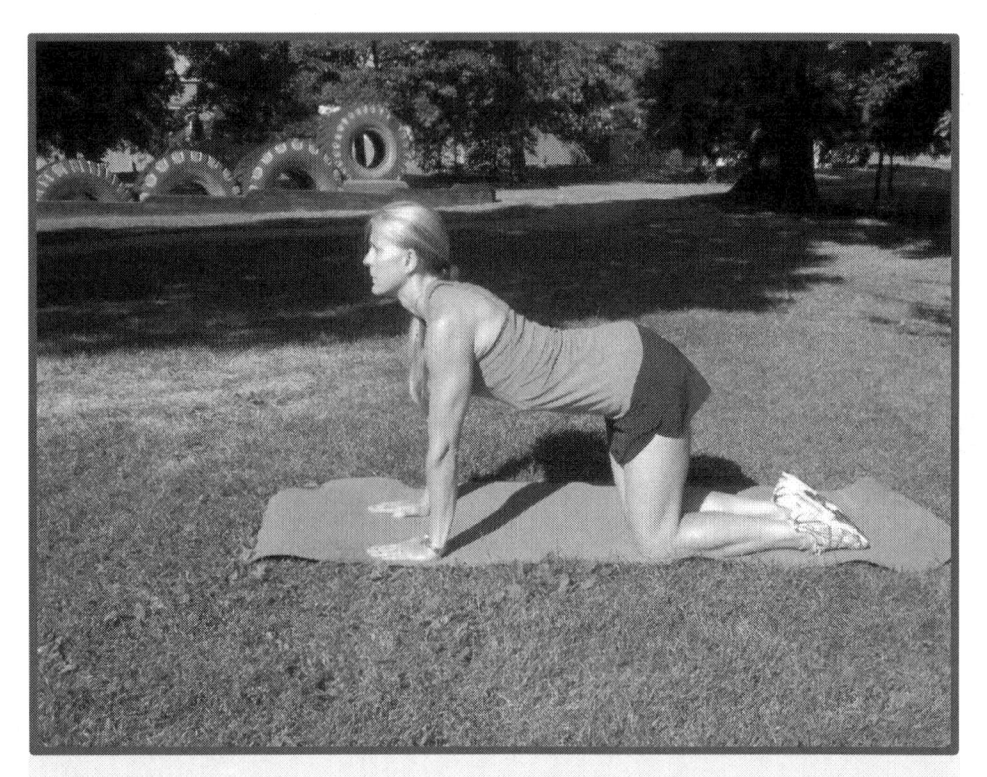

Special thanks to Lucy Hall -competitive body builder- of First Choice Fitness -www.firstchoicefitness.ca-

1. Position yourself on your hands and knees, with your head facing slightly forward. Inhale.

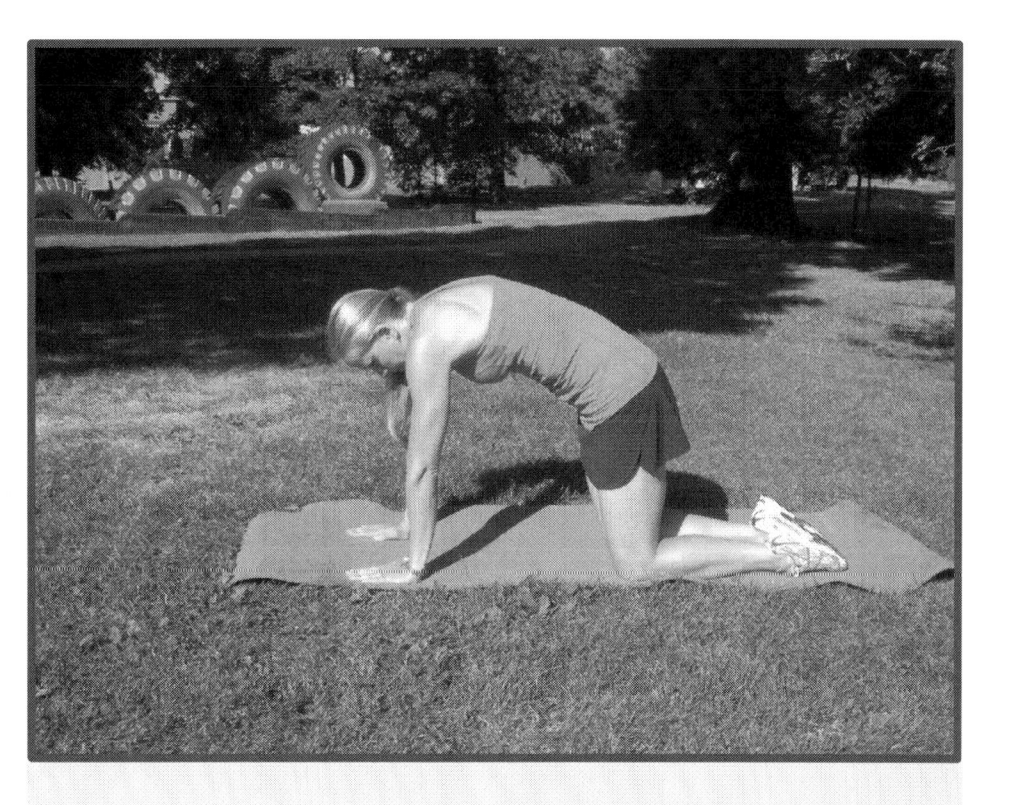

2. As you exhale, hunch your back like a cat, beginning at your tailbone and working your way up your spine to the back of your neck as you drop your head forward. Hold for two seconds.

3. Relax, inhale and return to the beginning position.

TORSO RAISE -Breaststroke Prep-

This is a great exercise to stretch the spine and strengthen the abdominal muscles. It is very useful for heavier people who feel pressure on their lungs when they try to perform sit-ups or crunches while lying on their backs. Most gyms do not recognize this and expect obese members to do crunches and sit-ups like an average person.

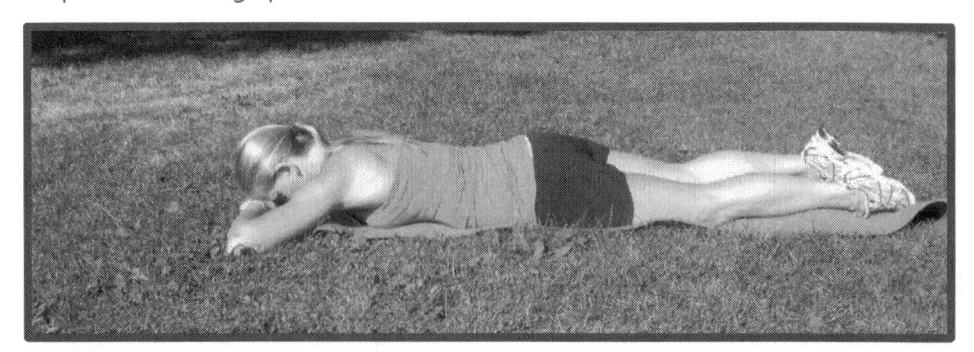

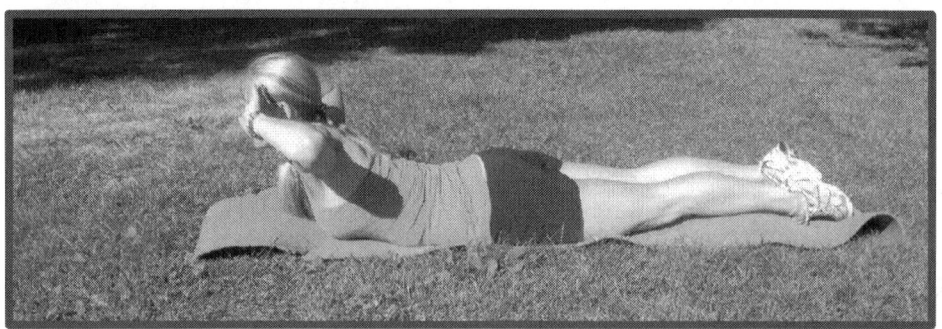

1. Start by lying face down on your mat, with your arms by your sides.

2. Keeping your legs on the mat, raise your head and torso off the mat. It is important not to hyperextend your chin, which tilts back the neck. Strive to keep your head straight and look at the floor, about a foot in front of you.

3. Repeat 4-12 times.

If you cannot perform a torso raise with your hands on your forehead, just start out with an easier variation.

Stage 1: Raise just your torso, with forearms on the mat Stage

2: Raise your torso with arms by your sides.

Stage 3: Raise your torso with the backs of your hands on your forehead and your elbows wide. When you can perform twelve of these, you can move on to the breaststroke exercise.

BREASTSTROKE

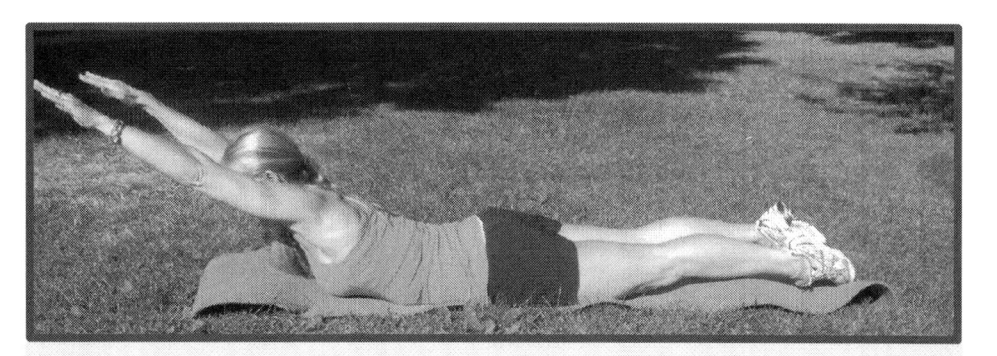

The breaststroke is performed lying face down on a mat.

1. Keeping your legs on the mat, raise your torso and hold the position.

2. With your torso still raised, extend your arms forward with your palms facing downward. Your arms should be by your ears.

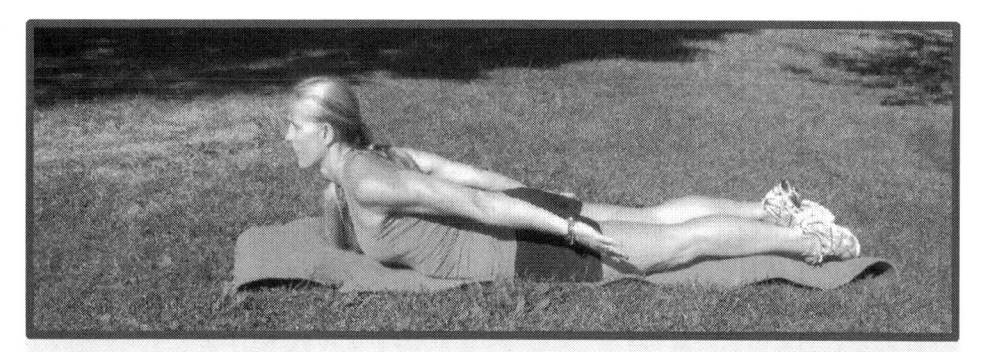

3. As you inhale, further raise your torso, as if you are performing a breaststroke. As you bring your hands alongside your body and extend your arms by your sides, keep your palms toward the mat. At the same time, bring your hands alongside your body and extend your arms by your thighs. Your palms remain facing the mat.

4. Exhale and reach forward and overhead again.

5. Repeat.

Perform 4-12 repetitions. Then perform the shell stretch.

SHELL STRETCH

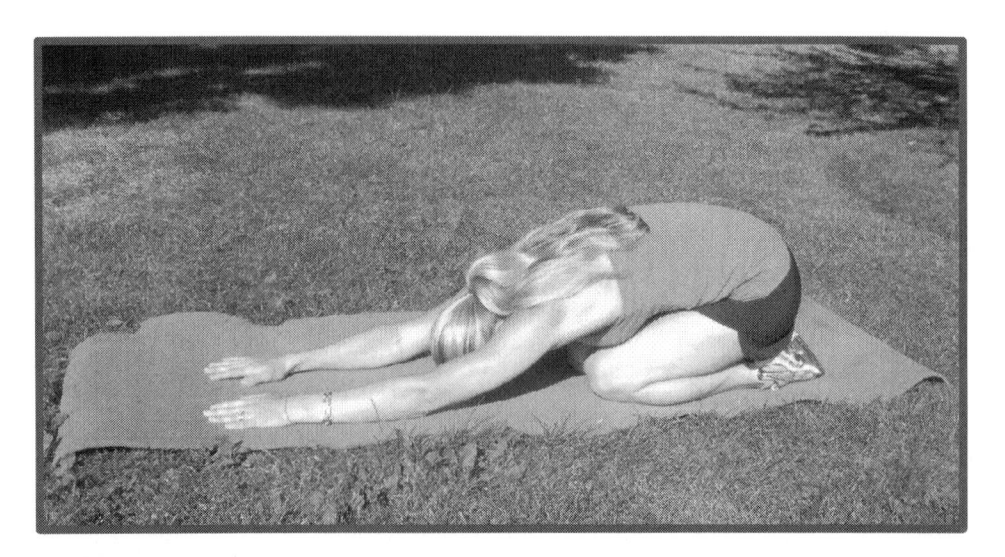

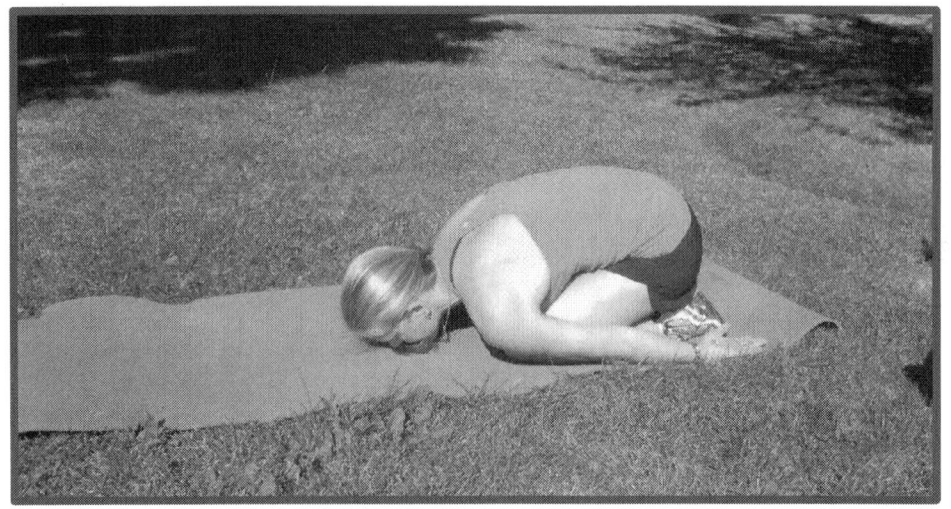

Otherwise known in yoga circles as the child or baby pose, the shell stretch is done immediately following back exercises. It is a comfortable position that takes pressure off your lower back. It also forces you to breathe deep into your lower lungs and abdominal area. This releases muscle tension and stimulates the digestive system.

ROLLING-LIKE-A-BALL

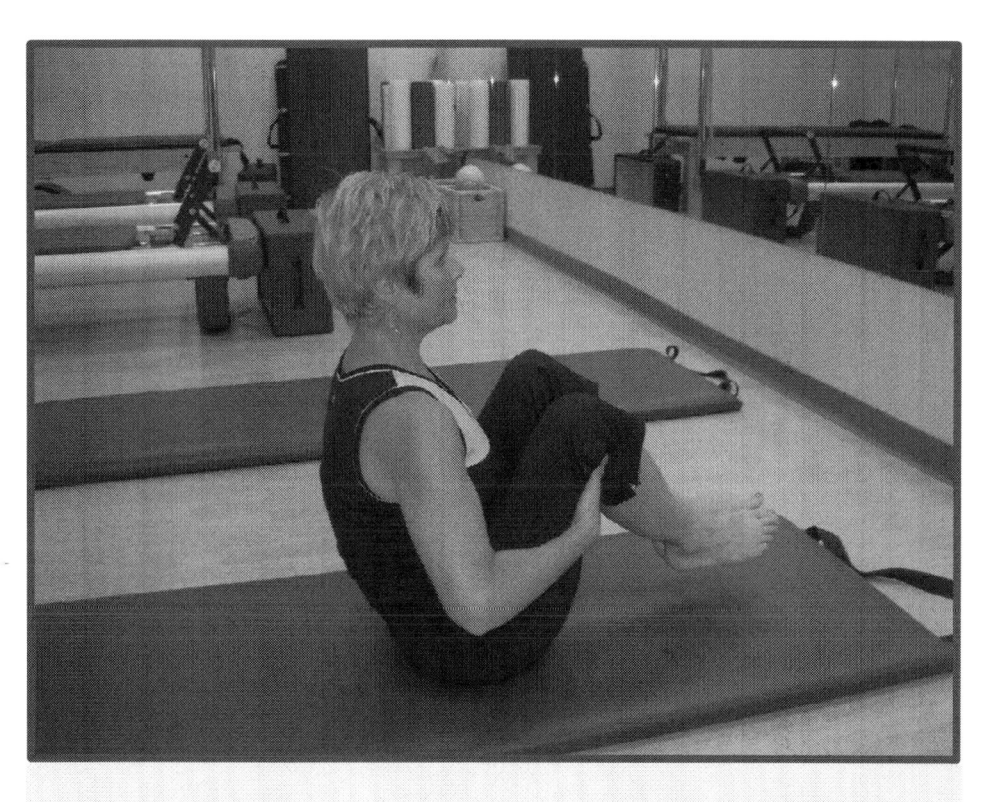

Special thanks to Pilates instructor and iron man competitor Monika Kriedmann-Bleckenwegner for modeling

This is a favorite of mine, as it strengthens the abdominal muscles while stretching the spine. The trick is to maintain a tight ball position while you are rocking back and forth. If you allow your back to flatten, you will often slam your back into the mat. Maintain that round back, like a rocking chair.

1. Start by balancing on your buttocks and "sit bones" -your pelvic bones just underneath your gluteus maximus or butt muscles-.

2. Place your hands on your hamstrings -beginners- or shins -intermediate- and hold your body in a tight ball.

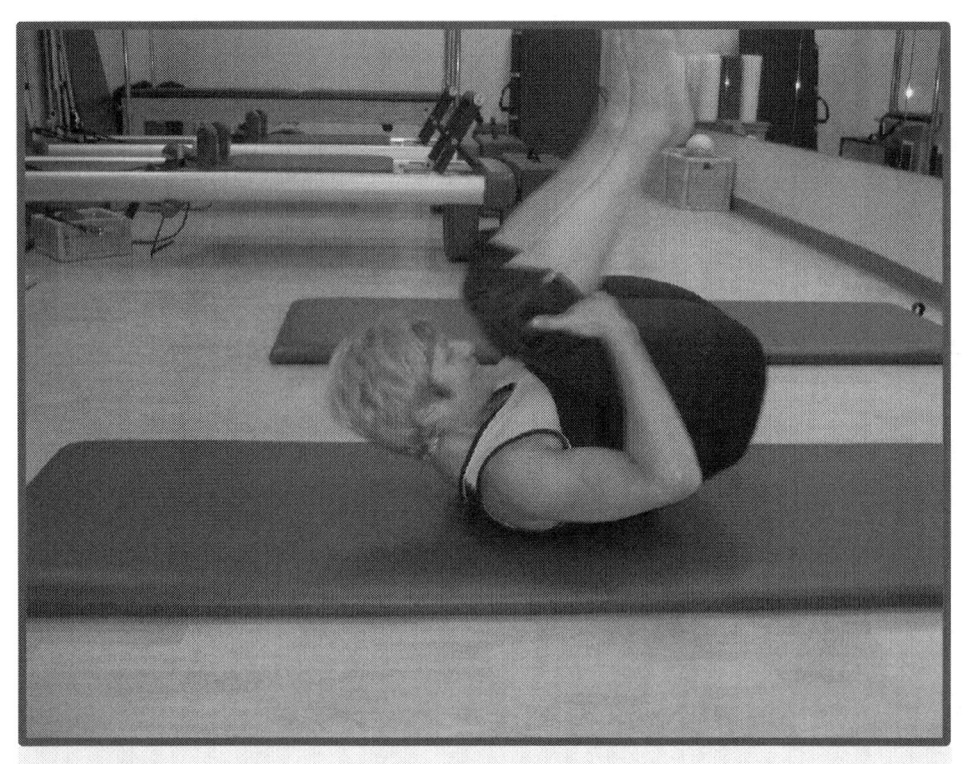

3. Rock backward until your shoulders -not the back of your head- are resting on the mat.

4. Then rock forward and shift hips, onto your sit bones, just before your feet touch the mat. Do not let your feet touch the mat.

5. Perform 4-12 repetitions. The slower the better.

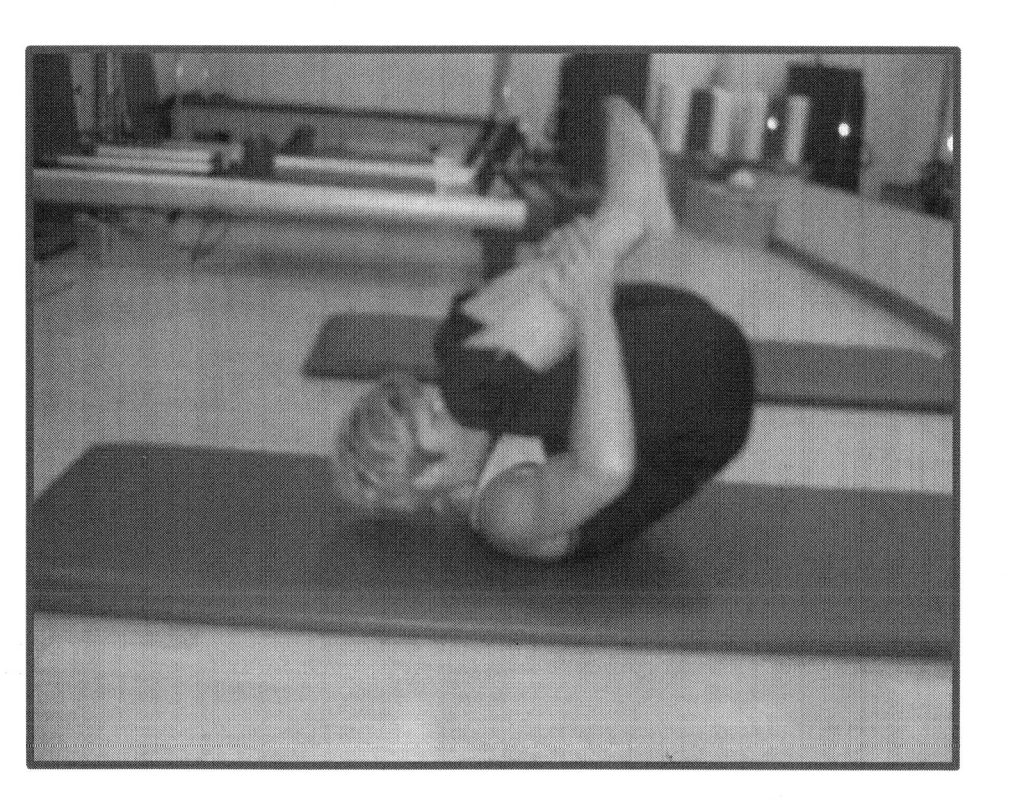

As you improve, you can move your hands to the outside of your shins and then your ankles.

It took me a few tries to get this exercise right. I initially banged the back of my head and landed flat on my back. The trick to doing this exercise properly is to keep your abdominal muscles tight, as if you are holding a quarter in your navel.

Some people are so tight in their lower backs that they require a pad or rolled up towel placed under the small of their back. As you get used to rolling over this "speed bump" pad, you can systematically unroll the towel until you are rolling like a ball on a flat surface. Do not despair if you do not get this movement on the first try.

I once trained two triathletes who could not do this movement until I used this rolled towel method. Each time that they rocked back and forth, I unraveled the towel a little bit. Within ten minutes they were doing the exercise almost perfectly. They had literally retrained their nervous systems to a new movement in a matter of minutes.

SINGLE-LEG CIRCLES

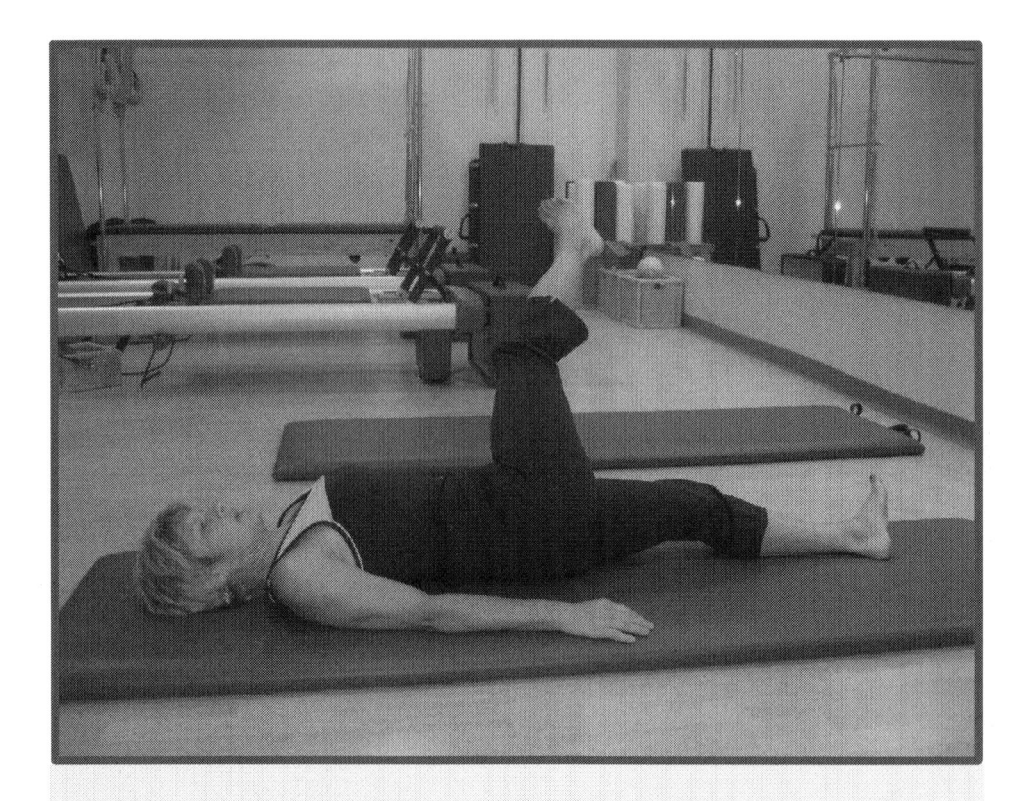

If there is an exercise that strengthens and tones that hard-to-reach, lower abdominal area, this is it. -Athletes and former pregnant women take note.-

1. Lie on your back with your arms by your sides.

2. With one leg prone on the mat, raise the other leg as straight as possible. Note: Some beginners will need to bend one or both legs due to muscle weakness.

3. Keeping the hips stabile, circle the upraised leg as wide as possible without allowing your hips to leave the mat, ten times each way. Repeat with other leg. A good way to maintain stability is to place a golf ball on your navel while circling your leg. If your hips become unstable, the ball will roll off.

4. Note: Bend your extended leg before lowering it to the mat. This takes pressure off your lower back.

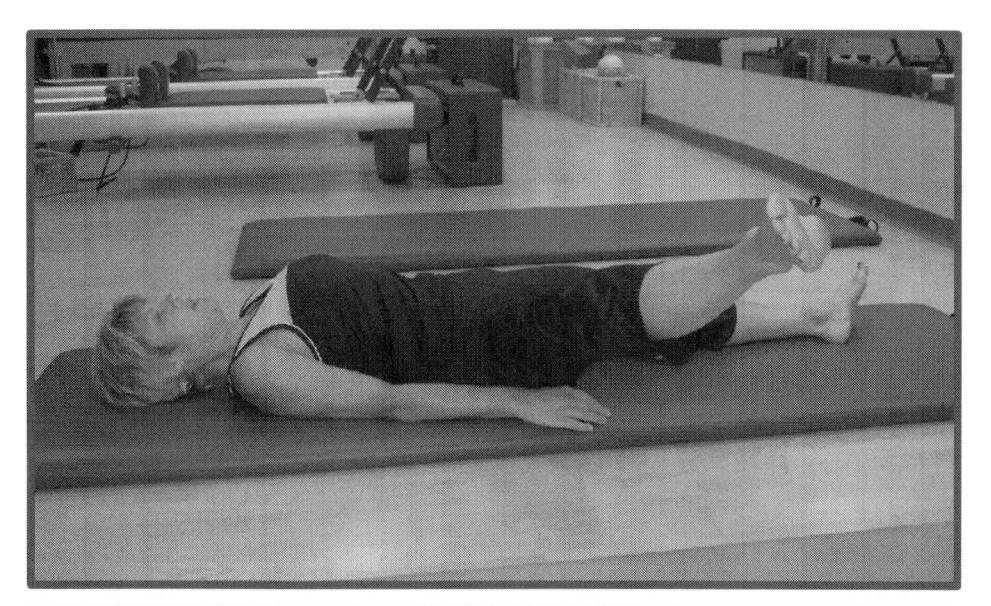

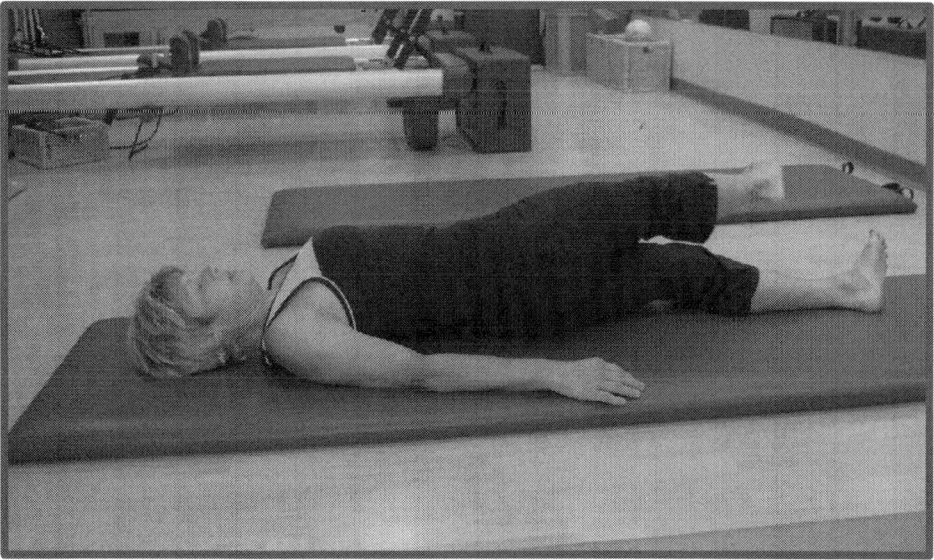

Avoid letting your hips leave the mat.

ROLL-UP

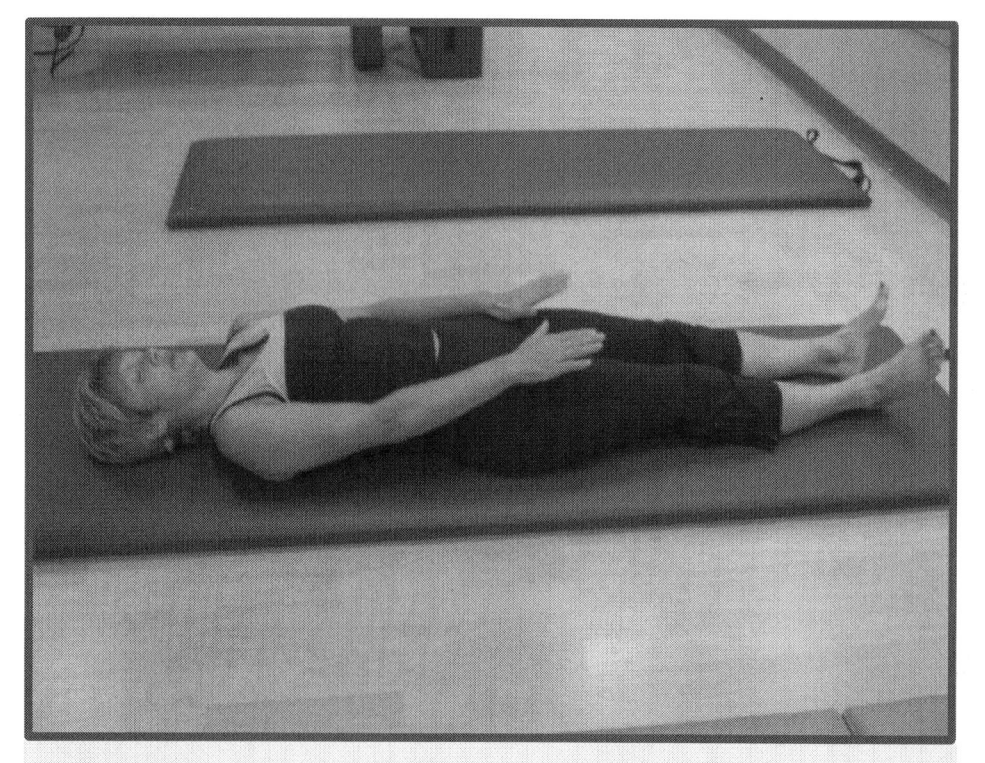

The roll-up is like a long sit-up except that you slowly roll forward. Here is how to perform it:

1. Lie on your back with your arms by your sides.

2. Inhale and reach upward the ceiling.

3. Exhale and place your hands down to your thighs.

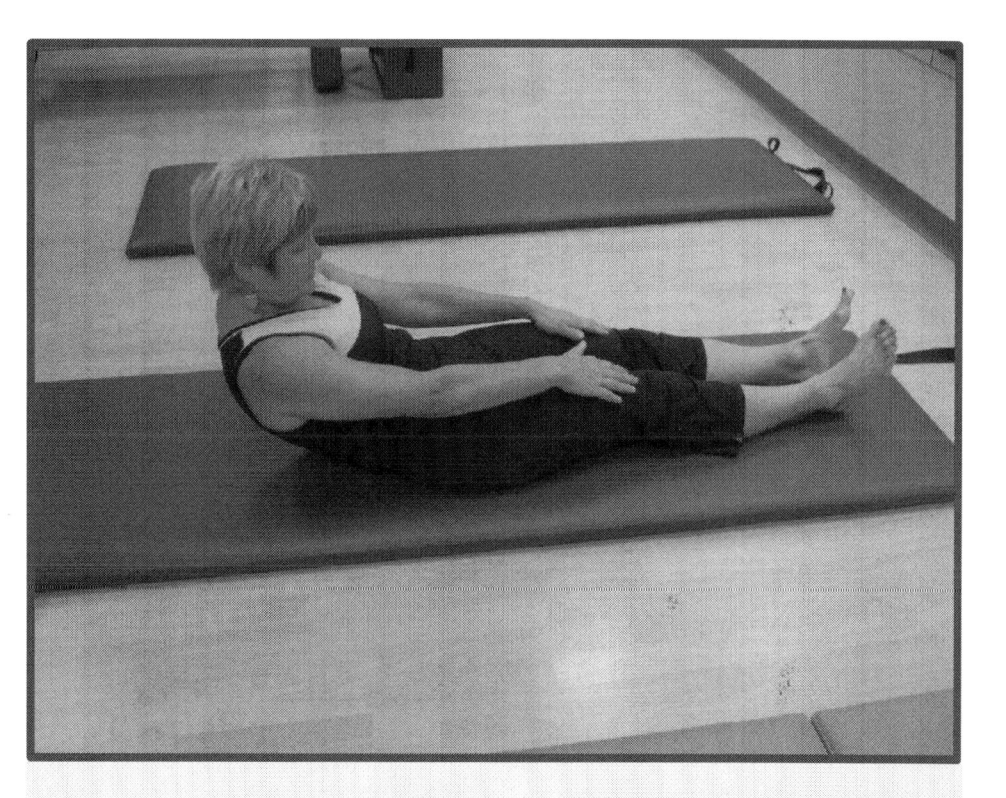

4. Bring your chin onto your chest and curl your upper body forward while reaching for your feet.

5. You must force the small of your back into the mat so that your cervical area -neck- leaves the mat, followed by the thoracic -upper and middle- area, and finally the lumbar -lower- portion of the spine leaves the mat. Try not to swing your arms forward to sit up.

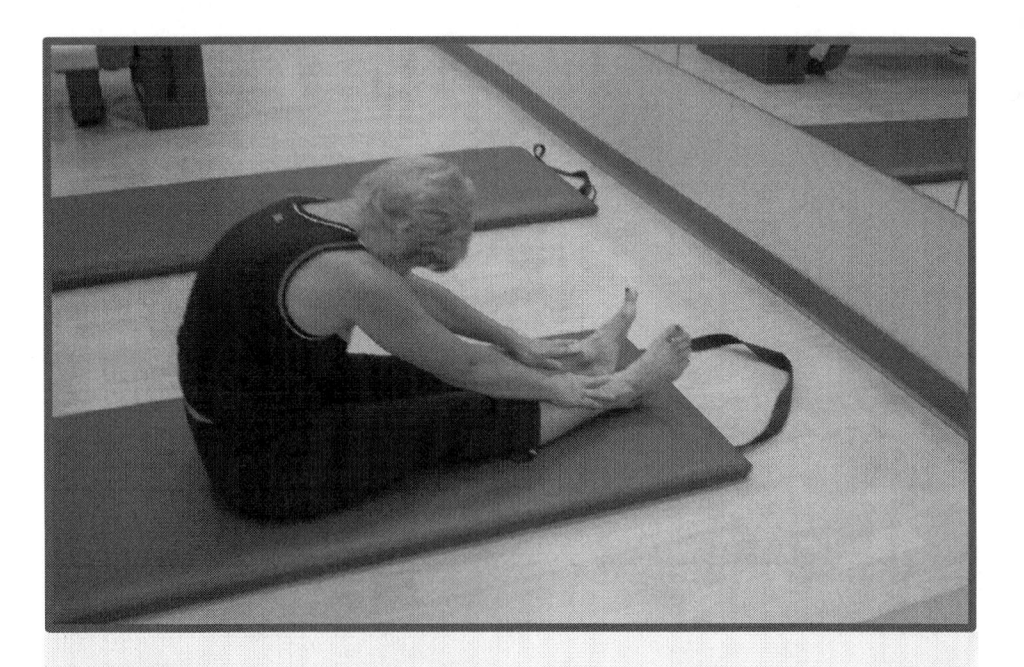

6. Exhale on the forward and inhale on the way back down.

7. Perform 4-12 repetitions.

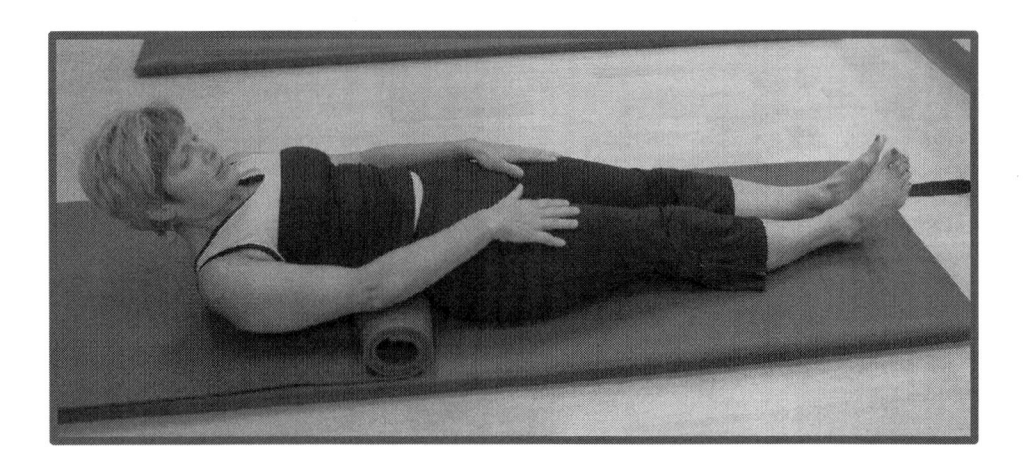

If, like some beginners, you cannot curl your upper body forward, you must really concentrate on forcing the small of your back into the mat. This can be assisted with the "speed bump" that was mentioned with the rolling-like-a-ball exercise. If you cannot sit up on your own, then roll up a towel and place it in the small of your back. You can also use bands anchored on your feet so that you can pull yourself up into a sitting position.

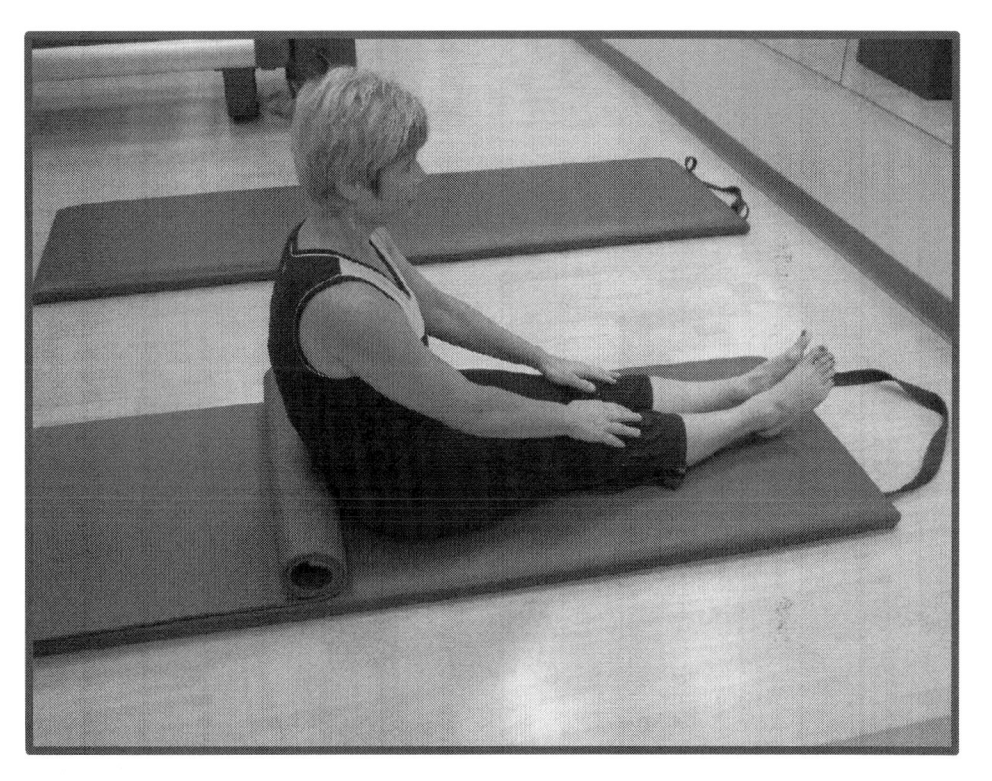

Another method to build up your strength and flexibility is to start from the sitting position and tuck the small of your back in while you roll down in reverse. Once you are prone, you can get back up into the straight-legged sitting position and lower yourself again.

SINGLE-LEG SEATED STRETCH

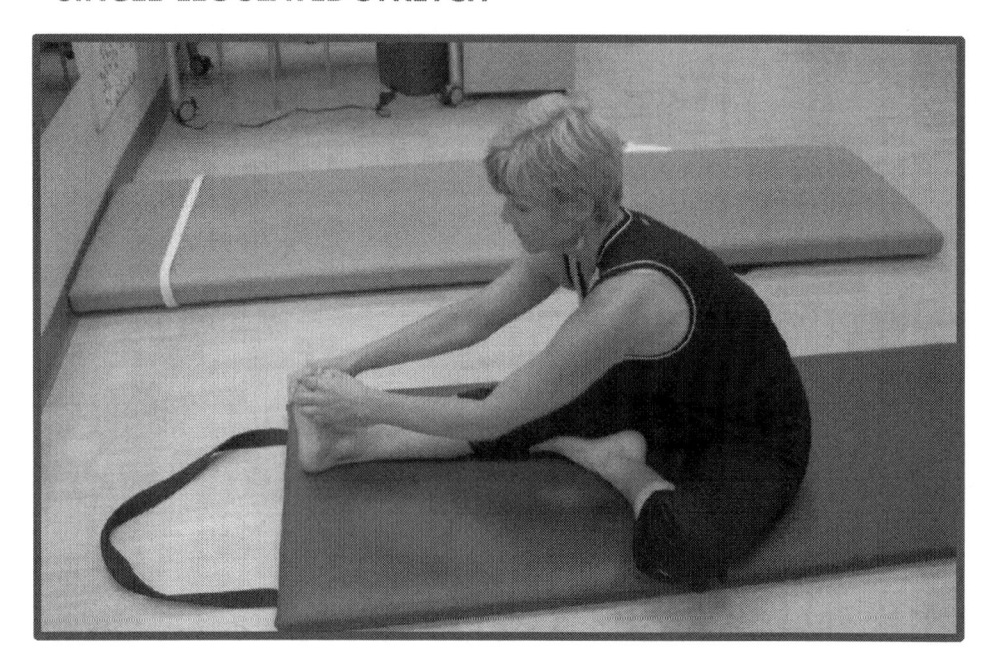

For the single-leg seated stretch, bring one foot into your groin and extend the other leg. Exhale as you extend both arms toward the foot of the extended leg and reach with your chin, not your forehead.

You perform the stretch this way for the following reasons:

- The exhaling helps release tension in your hamstrings.
- The "hands-free" pulling yourself forward activates your abdominal and hip flexor muscles while at the same time sending a signal to your lower back and hamstrings to relax.
- Reaching with the chin encourages stretching the lower back, while reaching with the forehead tends to stretch the upper back.
- Stretching one leg at a time reduces the risk of back injury.

No bouncing or yanking on your legs. When you use your abdominal and hip flexor muscles, without the use of your hands, you send a signal to your back muscles to release.

Now, as you pull yourself forward, exhale. You will often find that you can go a little further when you exhale instead of hold your breath.

SUSAN'S STORY

Susan grew up in rural Manitoba where the winter temperatures can drop below -40 °C. Later on, she moved to one of the coldest cities in North America, Winnipeg. There she worked in an office and taught fitness classes.

After her divorce, the mother of two boys was able to support her family by instructing fitness. Susan ran successful fitness and weight-loss bootcamps and instructed fitness classes for private gyms, school boards and even a drug rehabilitation program. She also freelanced as a consultant and fitness model.

Even though the -now- grandmother occasionally smoked and drank alcohol, she always disciplined herself to exercise. One of her favorite techniques for self-control was to make sure that she used exercise as a deterrent for certain vices. Whenever she smoked a cigarette, she would mark it down on her pack of cigarettes. Later on in the day, she performed five push-ups for every cigarette smoked.

Now past the half-century mark, Susan still exercises and remains strong and fit.

....

CHAPTER 04

TAKE A BREATH

TAKE A BREATH

Breathing. It is one of the most unappreciated, underutilized, unknown, forgotten, taken-for-granted and just plain ignored essential functions of the human body.

It's in our language: "Breathtaking," "catch my breath," "caught my breath," "It's all okay. Just breathe," "take a deep breath and calm down," "So scared, they couldn't breathe," "She was like a breath of fresh air."

Ancients, martial artists, athletes, singers and actors all know about the importance of breath. Focusing on breathing can triple your endurance, clear your mind, and improve your confidence and health.

Whether you are singing in an opera, breaking a stack of bricks, withstanding freezing cold water, exercising or instilling confidence, breathing techniques are almost always involved.

Let's take the typical office worker who spends most of their working day hunched in front of a computer. Before and after work, they spend an hour or so commuting in their car. Their slouched posture allows them about as much oxygen as a vegetable. There is no mystery here why they are often so fatigued at the end of the day that they flop down in front of the television set until bedtime.

When our sedentary desk jockeys do decide to exercise, they tend to stand out right away. Their struggled breathing is always heard in group fitness classes. They are usually at the back of the class panting and gasping for breath. If they can stick it out for the first three weeks, they normally start exhaling as they exert themselves.

THE BIG STAMINA BREATHING SECRET

So, here is the big breathing secret for improving your stamina: Breathe into your diaphragm and your lower lungs. Kids and animals breathe through their diaphragm without thinking. It is not until we get into adulthood that our bodies forget how to breathe deeply.

Does your body need a reminder?

Try running up and down a hill five times or jumping into cold water in

January. That will kick-start your natural breathing ability. You will most likely find that your body deliberately breathes deeply inhaling AND exhaling.

Which brings me to my next point: deep exhalation.

When you exhale deeply, you are expelling carbon dioxide along with several other toxic substances such as alcohol and ketones. It is accumulation of these toxic substances that can make us fatigued, NOT so much the lack of oxygen. This is why boxers snort, martial artists yell, and swimmers exhale fully.

Again, back to the fitness class scenario. In this case, it was kickboxing. In typical martial arts fashion, we exhale when we punch or kick. This expels the carbon dioxide and toxins while tightening the lower abdominal muscles. If you have ever seen some striking style -karate, tae kwon do, some forms of kung fu- martial artists without their shirts on, you will often notice the washboard abdominal muscles. The abdominal muscles are sometimes so defined that at the lower portion of the rib cage, near the obliques, it will look like an extra pair of ribs. -Do not worry. This is not our goal.-

Still another benefit of deep breathing is fat burning. As fat -consisting of carbon, hydrogen and oxygen- is broken down, it is exhaled as carbon dioxide. In a study in the British Medical Journal,[iv] 22 pounds -10 kg- of fat can turn into 18.5 pounds -8.4 kg- of carbon dioxide, which is exhaled. The remaining 3.5 pounds -1.6 kg- is water, which leaves the body through urine, tears and sweat.

ABDOMINAL BREATHING, COMPLETE BREATHING, AND THE CLEANSING BREATH

For this small chapter, we will cover abdominal breathing, complete breathing, and the cleansing breath. They are simple and can be learned through regular practice. Check out my breathing videos on www.2ndwindbodyscience.com.

ABDOMINAL BREATHING

This is vital for singers, actors and athletes.

1. Take a deep breath and exhale fully by letting your rib cage sink in. Next, tighten your abdominal muscles, forcing the air as much as you can.
2. Hold your breath. Do not inhale.
3. Force out a little more breath.
4. And a little more.
5. Relax and breathe.

Practice this until you can force out your breath, hold it, and force out THREE more short exhalations. You will often find that there are tightening abdominal muscles that you never even knew about. Start out slow so that you do not get muscle cramps or dizzy spells. If you do, then please consult your health professional.

You can do this exercise almost anywhere, including while driving a car or waiting at a bus stop or restaurant.

COMPLETE BREATH

This is where you can really get a rush of oxygen. So start out slow with this one.

1. Standing, sitting or lying down, exhale fully, as you did in the abdominal breathing. Squeeze the air out of your lower, middle and upper lungs.
2. Next, relax your lower abdomen and allow it to fill with air.
3. Then draw air into your middle lungs.
4. And finally, raise your rib cage and collarbone to draw air into your upper lungs.
5. Hold your breath for two seconds.
6. Exhale from your lower abdomen by tightening your abdominal muscles.
7. Then relax your middle rib cage.
8. Finally, relax your upper rib cage and collarbone.

Practice the complete breath no more than seven times in a row -some instructors recommend only once at a time- and no more than three times per day when you are starting out. I heard of a case where a yoga beginner practiced the complete breath fifty times several times a day. He ended up with a severe skin rash from a rush of toxins leaving his body. So, keep in mind that the complete breath can be a very powerful process.

CLEANSING BREATH

Note: Avoid the cleansing breath if you have high blood pressure.

The cleansing breath is usually performed during certain exercises -like the Pilates 100- or after exertion. I find that it can help calm me down after minor stresses, like traffic jams.

1. Standing, sitting or lying down, take a deep breath.
2. Purse your lips like you are blowing through a straw. It should be like blowing out candles from across the room.
3. Exhale like the abdominal breathing.
4. Relax, breathe normally, and repeat three times.

SUMMARY

- Deep breathing means more oxygen to your body and brain, making you more alert without stimulants.
- Deep breathing helps burn fat.
- Deep exhalation removes stale air and carbon dioxide and makes your body stronger and more stable.
- Deep breathing improves your stamina and overall health.

COLLEEN'S STORY

Colleen Wynia fought with mild depression from an early age.

"I was hurting and I did not know it," explained the fit fifty-one-year-old. "I had lost my dad and cousin to cancer and other loved ones to cancer, heart disease, Alzheimer's, seizures, drug addiction and suicide."

"I began diving into answers to recovery and ultimately prevention. Introspection led me to realize that depression was merely a symptom of much deep-rooted issues. This started me on a personal healing journey through exercise, nutrition, breathwork, massage, intuitive readings, meditation, and spirituality. One of my mentors was a spiritual medium and bodyworker who worked for the Vancouver Police Department helping them solve homicide cases. Of course, back then, it was rare to consult a spiritual medium. Our work together led me to train for three and a half years with Shamballa Trainings, a community that combined teachings of Western psychology and counsel with Eastern traditions that embody the body, mind, and heart."

"I learned that one could study and essentially hold a Master's degree in psychology or years of mindset training, but the true transformation of healing is revealed through the body. That the body ultimately absorbs and retains past life memories, childhood negative experiences, and life traumas that may condition the body into symptoms that mimic physical dis-ease states or mental health issues long-term, such as depression."

"As I progressed with integrating a conscious, connected breathing practice known as rebirthing, my own pain appeared to leave my pain body. The breathwork alone provided me the lift I needed to face life and move forward each day."

"It's been twenty-five years since that painful year when my father Gerry and cousin Rob transitioned within nine months of each other. I thank them every day for their loving presence and the spiritual cheerleaders they have become. I now recognize and deeply appreciate the •death triggers' that redirected my life to teach spiritual practices and modalities that ease pain and inspire new life. I've experienced the great gift of helping hundreds of women, men and youth transform their pain into emotional freedom to live happier, healthier, longer lives with a sense of purpose. I embraced the role as a •Reset Your Vibe' Energy Coach and Spiritual Intuitive."

"To sustain my peace of mind and continue the internal healing, exercise is a huge thing at the end of the day," Colleen remarks. "Maintaining a high level of fitness and fueling my body with whole food supplementation is key to my well-being."

Colleen's exercise primarily consists of elliptical cardio training, Bikram yoga and Body-Weight Exercise -BWE-. Hiking up and down North Vancouver's Grouse Mountain and other steep trails truly fuels Colleen's joy and connection to nature. Much to the dismay of her friends, Colleen insists on walking by herself at night. "I feel that I can recover from the day and channel my thoughts and emotions in the tranquility of the night. It is so calming and peaceful."

One night, while crossing a wooden bridge, Colleen was surprised by a black bear walking toward her, eye to eye. "The bear was heading straight toward me. I stepped out of his path and was amazed how nonchalant Mr. Bear was as he kept on cruising and turned down an adjacent path with clear intention," she laughs.

As for nutrition, she eats mostly vegetarian and enjoys stir-fried tofu and organic raw spinach in her daily vegan protein smoothies. She also consumes two powerhouse whole-food beverage supplements known as Mangosteen, the Queen of Fruits of Thailand, and moringa oleifera, commonly grown in India and parts of Asia. The botanicals, which have anti-cancer properties, have kept her free from colds and flu for years.

What ignites Colleen to get up each day, even when feeling the occasionally low mood, is her drive to make a difference in the lives of others, to help them discover emotional freedom.

"There is no other option," the fit, blonde businesswoman insists. "I am either here for a purpose or I am not. To have the life that I want, I show people ways to transform their experiences of loss, grief and pain while gaining deeper levels of self-trust, self-direction and self-confidence."

Colleen's website is www.ColleenWynia.com

••

CHAPTER 05

EATING, ENERGY AND ENTERTAINMENT

EATING, ENERGY AND ENTERTAINMENT

When I was around eight years old, I read about how different cultures of the world ate. Their diets ranged from a cattle blood and milk mixture of the Maasai tribesman in Africa to the fish and rice in Japanese culture to the corn-based diet of Guatemala. I also learned, much to my young mind's disgust, that the people of France ate over 600 million snails per year! Yet French people, with their diets high in fat, bread, tobacco and wine, also enjoy good health and low rates of heart disease.[v]

Even as a child, I often wondered why many of these traditional cultures seemed to have better health than North Americans. This was back in the mid-sixties to early seventies when the big cholesterol scare condemned fat, milk and meat and drove up wheat consumption. A decade later, I woke up to the fact that the low-fat, low-protein, high-sugar and processed foods were keeping me sick, scrawny and underweight.

Ignoring the national food guidelines, education boards, dieticians, and even the nutrition department of the University of Manitoba -and other so-called experts-, I read up on nutrition and sought out super healthy people. After following their advice on high-energy eating, my allergies disappeared, and I became stronger, calmer and could think more clearly.

The basis of high-energy eating is getting the needed nutrients and keeping the blood sugar stable. -Sugar and insulin are mentioned in Chapter 2, Happy Hormones.- This is the basis of diets like the popular keto, Atkins, Scarsdale and glycemic index diets. Low-index foods -glycemic rating of 55 or below-, such as meat, butter, lentils, chickpeas and whole grains, maintain a stable level of blood sugar. High-glycemic foods -rating of 70 or more-, such as white bread, white rice, white potatoes, most fruit and processed breakfast cereals, cause large fluctuations in the blood sugar. -See Canadian Diabetes Association for a more detailed list: https://www.diabetes.ca/ managing-my-diabetes/tools---resources/the-glycemic-index--gi-.-

Fact: Stable blood sugar maintains energy levels, supports the immune

Breakfast -if eaten at all-	Cereal, waffles and/or toast, orange juice and coffee
Break	Donut or muffin, coffee
Lunch	Salad with dressing, ham sandwich and flavored yogurt
Break	Apple, coffee
Supper	Pasta noodles, tomato sauce, boiled potatoes, carrot sticks, apple pie
Snack	Pastry

system and helps control the appetite. You have probably experienced a drop in energy or thinking ability after consuming a heavy, starchy meal or sugary treats. This is often your body reacting to the sugar and dumping large amounts of insulin into your bloodstream. This surge of insulin causes your blood sugar to drop and makes you more vulnerable to fatigue, stress and illness. Along with fatigue and brain fog, you might also feel weak and experience muscle tremors.

Here is a typical eating pattern for many North Americans.

Breakfast *-if eaten at all-*	2-3 eggs boiled or fried, dark rye toast, butter, bowl of steel-cut or pressed oats
Break	Humus and crackers or high-protein smoothie
Lunch	Tuna salad with balsamic dressing, chicken strips
Break	Herbal tea
Supper	Lean hamburger, stir-fried vegetables, oven roasted yams, baked apple
Snack	Turkey strips, oatmeal crackers

As you can see a mile away, this eating routine is packed with sugar, which would leave the average person groggy and reaching for coffee or another sugar boost.

PROTEINS	FATS	VEGETABLES	GRAINS	FRUITS	MISC.
Beef Chicken	Butter Almond butter	Green vegetables -broccoli, cabbage, celery, lettuce, Brussel sprouts, etc.- Orange/red vegetables -carrots, yams, beets- Bean sprouts	Brown rice	Apples	"Designer shakes" -protein drinks- Protein bars
Turkey Fish	Olive oil Sesame oil		Millet Oatmeal Couscous	Apricots Pears	
Eggs Tofu	Flaxseed oil Cashew butter		Kasha Kamut	Berries	

THE FOODS THAT SUPPORT YOU

In this section, I highlight key foods and food groups that you can use to build a more stable meal plan, such as the one below:

You can save time by cooking most of your meals one or two nights a week -e.g. Sunday- and then packaging the cooked food in wraps and/ or Tupperware. Usually the food preparation takes less than forty minutes, especially if you use your oven and bake everything. This early preparation can feed you for a couple of days afterward. It saves time and money in the long run.

Protein	50 g -usually 1 gram per kilogram of body weight-
Vitamins	5-10 times the minimum recommended daily allowance, e.g. 800 IU of vitamin E; 10,000 IU of vitamin A

MINERALS

Calcium	1,200 mg
Magnesium	600 mg
Zinc	30 mg

EATING FOR ENERGY

High protein, some fats -fish oils- and diets high in complex carbohydrates can boost your energy in a week or less. Except in rare situations, you should be able to eat the following:

By eating nutrient-rich foods, you save more money and give yourself a greater energy return than if you eat low-value foods such as donuts or cake. -By the way, beer and nacho chips are not food groups.-

If you are not satisfied with the foods on the given list, look up other foods in a reputable nutrition book like *Nutrition Almanac*[vi]. You might be surprised at what you thought were nutritious foods. For instance, broccoli contains more potassium than bananas, and black currants have over twice the vitamin C as oranges.

NUTRIENTS FOR HEALTHY SKIN[vii]

To build healthy skin and protect your skin from stress, pollutants and toxins, your body requires water, protein, vitamins, minerals and fresh air.

HEALTHY FATS

"You have too much fat in your diet," the overweight woman said to the fit-looking woman.

I overheard this conversation while I was standing in line at the grocery store. The overweight woman gave quite a lecture about fat to a clearly fitter and healthier woman. Being the eager researcher -and a bit of a snoop-, I looked at their food selections.

The fit woman's selections were meat, vegetables, butter and 6% fat yogurt. The overweight woman's choices were fruit -high sugar-, bread, chips and frozen French fries. Enough said.

The danger in fat is not in its high caloric value -nine kilocalories per gram-. It is dangerous when it is processed, like hydrogenated fat -trans fat-, or becomes rancid -oxidized-.

Polyunsaturated fats -like vegetable oils-, which were all the rage during the big fat scare of the 1970s, become rancid faster than saturated fats -like butter-. Much safer are monounsaturated fats like cold-pressed olive oil. Fresh, cold-pressed oils are very beneficial -e.g. may reduce inflammation in the joints and brain-. However, they require proper storage and have a short shelf life once they are exposed to air.

There is an experiment where rats that were fed polyunsaturated fats made more errors in a maze than rats fed saturated fats.[viii] The theory is that polyunsaturated fats going rancid affected the rats' brains, while the saturated fats did not go rancid as quickly and therefore did not affect the rats' performances.

Another fat fact is that most saturated fats contain fat-soluble vitamins, such as A, D, E and K. These vitamins are important for the skin, mood, eyesight and blood clotting. Vitamin D deficiency can cause susceptibility to brittle bones, rickets and muscle spasms. Even bouts of depression, such as "the winter blues" -from lack of sunlight-, can be attributed to a vitamin D deficiency.

Despite the rants about "that bad saturated fat," grass-fed butter is a good choice for brain and body health and has many benefits that include the following:

- Contains vitamins A, D, E, K2 and B12
- Contains Conjugated Linoleic Acid -CLA-, which may reduce heart

disease. CLA was very popular among women fitness trainees for mood and weight maintenance.

- May reduce inflammation in joints and brain
- Is healthier than grain-fed butter or margarine

FRIENDLY INTESTINAL BACTERIA

Bacteria have been living in human digestive tracts in symbiotic existence for thousands of years. Usually, we have a good working relationship. The good bacteria can help us by

- Improving our immune systems
- Preventing harmful bacteria from infecting us
- Providing vitamins
- Breaking down and helping us absorb food

These bacteria can also inhibit or promote weight gain and improve mood. Researchers biologist Jeffery Gordon of Washington University in St. Louis and graduating student Peter Turnbaugh were able to decrease or promote weight in mice by changing the mice's intestinal bacteria. They found that both thin humans and mice had different bacteria -known as Bacteroidetes- than obese humans and mice -Firmicutes-. It was also found that within twenty-four hours of consuming high-fat, high-sugar food, the obese -Firmicutes- bacteria increased and their host mice became fatter.

Without changing your caloric intake, you can actually become leaner and healthier -and calmer- by adding beneficial bacteria to your diet. Examples are sauerkraut, kimchi, kefir, miso soup, plain yogurt and probiotics.

WHAT TO AVOID

When you work hard at exercising and eating right, you can sometimes treat yourself with various junk and non-foods. But for the most part, you really want to avoid certain substances, especially the white carbohydrates. The big six substances to avoid are: sugar, wheat, milk, alcohol, caffeine and nicotine.

WHITE SUGAR

One of the most damaging sweet-tasting substances overconsumed in the

North American diet is white sugar, also known as sucrose or table sugar.

Not only is it highly addictive, white sugar also depletes the body of B vitamins, magnesium, chromium and other minerals. Sugar is also responsible for tooth decay, nervousness, hypoglycemia -low blood sugar-, allergies and mood swings.[ix] Depressed people are often suffering from low blood sugar and vitamin B deficiencies.[x] The overconsumption of sugar inhibits the immune system, especially when it is consumed just before sleep.[xi]

Heavy sugar consumption also causes glycation, which can dry out your skin. So, think about that before you eat another donut.

Here are some rules to keep in mind about eating sugar:

- Always eat some protein before consuming sugar. -This slows down the absorption of sugar.-
- Avoid eating sugar within 1.5 hours of sleeping. -It inhibits the growth hormone for body repair and fat burning.-
- It's better to eat small amounts throughout the day instead of large amounts at a time.

WHITE FLOUR

Bleached wheat flour is the main ingredient in the paste for paper-mache. So, imagine your stomach trying to break down paste.

White flour has almost all of the food value removed and is difficult to digest. For the most part, it gives you a full feeling without much benefit. Heavy white flour eaters typically have bloated stomachs and thin arms and legs.

Though it is in most fast food, you can avoid it. For example, it is OK to eat a hamburger and toss the bun.

PASTEURIZED MILK

Most people lose the lactase enzyme after the age of two, so it is unnatural to consume milk after early childhood, human or otherwise. Maybe you can drink gallons of pasteurized milk with no allergic reactions. If so, try going without it for five days. You will probably go through a bit of a withdrawal but feel much better for it in the long run.

If you are concerned about a lack of calcium, keep in mind that most of the world does well without milk and has lower rates of osteoporosis than North America. There are many sources of calcium in foods like fish, green vegetables, beans, bone broth and calcium supplements. -I prefer the 2:1 calcium-magnesium tablets.-

Except for some fermented dairy products like cheese, yogurt and kefir, I have consumed very little milk for the past forty years. My bones have not shattered, nor have my teeth fallen out. My sinuses are much clearer than they were in my high school years, and I am sick less often.

ALCOHOL

Alcohol is a popular drug of choice. It goes great with meals and social gatherings. Some forms, such as red wine, claim to have health benefits including antioxidants and anti-inflammatories. Personally, I have enjoyed good quality beer and wine in Europe and Asia with few side effects. In some circles, one or two drinks per day is considered healthy.

Overconsumption and habitual drinking is another matter. Besides depleting vitamins and minerals, alcohol can lower blood sugar levels and give rise to a host of physical and emotional problems. Too much alcohol can deplete the appetite, so the drinker will tend to stop eating and neglect their health. Also, cheaper forms of alcohol contain additives like formaldehyde.

Following are a few rules regarding alcohol:

- Eat something with fat and protein before drinking.
- Spread out your drinks with juice or water.
- Choose good quality alcohol.

There are six basic reactions to alcohol, which you can learn about in my books *Reduce Your Alcohol Craving* and *Simple Secrets to Handle Your Alcohol Better: Student's Edition*.

CAFFEINE

You might notice how heavy coffee drinkers are often tired and irritable, especially when they do not get their regular caffeine fix.

Caffeine is in many food products, including coffee, chocolate and green tea. While it can keep people alert, it can also increase blood sugar levels and exhaust the adrenal glands. When the adrenaline hormones become depleted, energy levels lower. As mentioned before, these adrenaline hormones are meant to take you into old age. Heavy coffee consumption increases the cortisol hormone, which can increase body fat and blood pressure, depress your mood and cause muscle weakness.

Take caffeine only in small amounts.

NICOTINE

Nicotine can increase concentration in some people. For this reason, it has often been used in small amounts during study and certain spiritual ceremonies. Personally, I have smoked natural tobacco from a peace pipe during a sweat lodge ceremony and found that the tobacco was neither addictive nor irritating like the commercial brands.

Processed tobacco is another matter. Being around heavy smokers for the first two decades of my life weakened my lungs and probably contributed to my early bouts of pneumonia. Processed tobacco is full of nickel, lead, copper and tar, which deplete nutrients, lower the immune system and contribute to the formation of arterial plaque. It is also an expensive habit.

Nicotine cure: Some former smokers have reported kicking their habit by chewing small amounts of the herb lobelia. While not a smoker, I have noticed that many expensive formulas contain some form of lobelia. So, if you are smoker, you can save both your health and your bank account by giving it a try.

EATING AND ENTERTAINMENT

Keep in mind that the best foods in the world could be rejected by your body if you do not like it or are in a foul mood. You are probably better off eating a hotdog with good friends than an expensive dinner with people whom you despise.

This brings us to the culture of eating. Most cultures take eating as a happy event. Hunting, gathering, shopping, cooking and sharing food has always been a social activity. You can even make an event out of a simple meal. I have had great times with friends and relatives making different dishes. The kitchen can be a great place to hang out -or get yelled at-.

And if you find food preparation to be a necessary, boring task, you might want to learn to cook better. Do you want to improve your health and social life? Learn to cook tastier meals and attend cooking classes. Cooking and entertaining friends is a wonderful skill. Many a successful business meeting or date has involved eating a good meal. In fact, it often calms down hostilities.[xii]

Eating with good company is good for your mood and will often improve your digestion. Even with a busy schedule, it is highly recommended to have at least one good, sit-down, two-hour meal per week with friends and loved ones. It can do wonders for your health and mood.

Remember that you are human. The occasional carrot cake, glass of wine or cigarette is not going to kill you -immediately-.

CHAPTER 06

FUNCTIONALLY FIT

FUNCTIONALLY FIT

Are you the type to practice an hour daily of Zumba or swimming? Or lifting weights? Or how about daily yoga and boating on weekends? Or do you do your own shopping and enjoy gardening?

This is exactly what many people in their forties, fifties, sixties and beyond are doing.

Exercise, movement and activity all promote blood and oxygen flow, clear the mind and improve digestion, strength, bone density and mood. Exercise has been labeled "the fountain of youth." As mentioned in Chapter 2, Happy Hormones, exercise also improves the production of hormones. Why would you NOT want to feel better, be more productive, be able to move, stretch, work and play with your grandchildren?

Note: The bones of a sixty-year-old woman who weight trains can be denser and stronger than those of a twenty-year-old woman who does not exercise.

Hopefully, by now you've also fully adopted or at least practiced some of the posture exercises. If yes, good on you! If no, please take two minutes now and try at least one of them.

Finally, you probably already know the value of a good warm-up. Something as simple as a jog around the block, ten minutes of dancing or warming up to music, or riding a bike or even stationary bike. Please do this. At sixty-two years of age, I sometimes skip this part and often pay for it.

TRAINING

Training is the serious part of fitness. This is where you aim for results, so no messing around. We get in there, have a good time, and get the job done.

You want to have a body that can perform a wide range of movements. This is the beauty of many body-weight exercises. The movements are, for the most part, natural and functional. Examples are picking up and carrying a bag of groceries -or squirming infant-, lifting objects overhead, running to catch a bus, touching the floor, dancing, and the classic "springing out of bed" in the morning.

So, what we are looking for is strength, endurance, balance and flexibility. If that sounds like a big bill to fill, don't worry. It can be done if you approach it intelligently.

END STATE

When you train to improve yourself, you should have a good reason and some kind of end state or goal. For instance, for years I used to just run, work out and practice martial arts because I enjoyed it. But when a race, competition or military course came up, I trained more seriously for results. There was no time wasting or excess socializing. I had to be ready for that race, competition or course. Failure meant embarrassment and a whole lot of pain for nothing. A little bit of why you are training can really focus your energy and personal drive.

Casually just wanting to "tone up" is not nearly as motivating as exercising because you want to be ready for a wedding -maybe your own-, climbing Mt. Rainier, ballroom dancing, enjoying a sailing trip, applying for a job or completing a 10 km run.

You will note that I did not mention burning calories, losing pounds and inches, reducing back pain or lowering blood pressure. These are side benefits of exercise, NOT the main goal. Scales and measuring tapes are annoying distractions when you should be focusing on performance and how you feel. The cosmetics and other health benefits will come. So let's get started.

ENDURANCE TRAINING

Cardiovascular -cardio- exercise was very popular in the 1970s, when there was a marked increase in heart and lung disease. This gave way to huge government fitness campaigns and the 1.5 mile run Cooper test. The rampant heart disease was probably more from labor-intensive work being replaced by automation and people's general laziness. Couple those with heavy tobacco, alcohol and processed food consumption, and hello, heart disease.

Cardio-like activities, on the other hand, are the spice of life. Long distance running, swimming, cycling, kayaking, hiking and most sports usually put the participant outside in the fresh air. Cardio or endurance activities will almost always put you in a good mood with an endorphin high.

"But I hate running!" or "I'm too embarrassed!" are typical excuses that I have heard over the decades. This might spring from being shamed in gym class, sports or the military. Nonetheless, you are denying your natural ability to move and experience that boost of oxygen and endorphins. No one says that you have to look like a superstar to get on a bike, walk, fly a kite or jog around the park. The beauty of cardio training is that it is cheap and relatively easy to do anywhere and with anyone.

The shortcoming of endurance -cardio- exercises is that they often do not build bone density, muscle and the antiaging effects of your anabolic metabolism. Strength or resistance training can fill that bill.

RESISTANCE TRAINING

Resistance training is like life: There always seems to be resistance against what you are trying to accomplish. But through this resistance, we build strength and resilience.

Resistance training builds bone density and activates your body's rebuilding mechanisms and hormonal system. While aerobic exercise builds endurance and makes you feel good, it usually does not have the same antiaging results as resistance training does. Resistance or strength training, such as weightlifting, tears down muscle so that your body rebuilds itself.

Weightlifting is a reliable method to build lean muscle, burn fat and increase your anabolism. Free weights are superior to machines as they demand more body control, core engagement and balance. If you look around any gym, you will usually see the fitter people lifting free weights.

It's best to start weight training with light weights and instruction. It is always better to use strict technique for fewer repetitions than sloppy technique for more repetitions. Start with one and work up to three sets.

As you become stronger and more experienced, you might advance to heavier weights and different reps and sets.

The following are lightweight exercises that have seen good results.

LIGHTWEIGHT RESISTANCE TRAINING EXERCISES

REVERSE LUNGE

The reverse lunge is great for building leg strength AND balance.

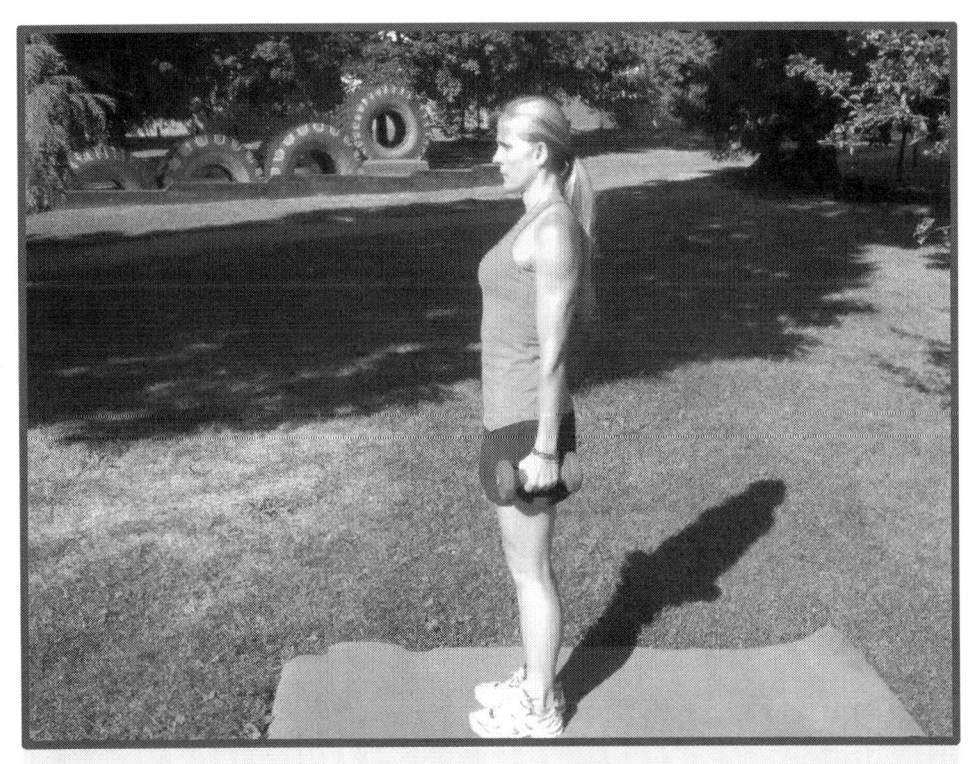

Special thanks to fitness model Lucy Hall, professional bodybuilder and grandmother.

1. Stand with your feet shoulder-width apart -with or without a weight in each hand-.

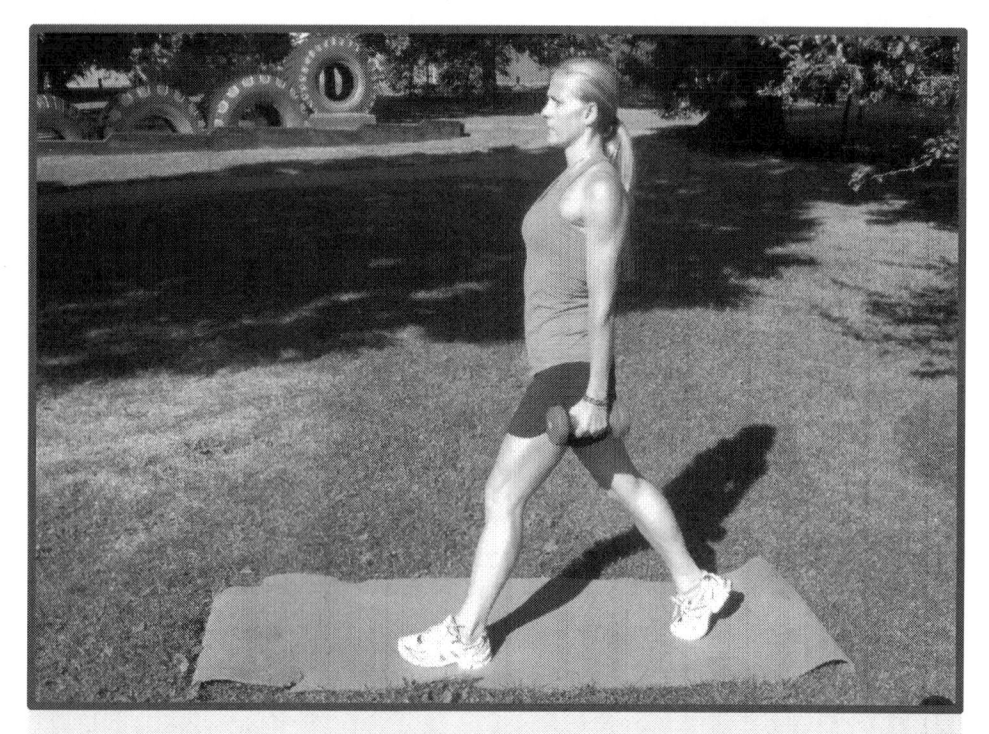

2. Step back with one leg, about 2.5 feet to a meter to the rear.

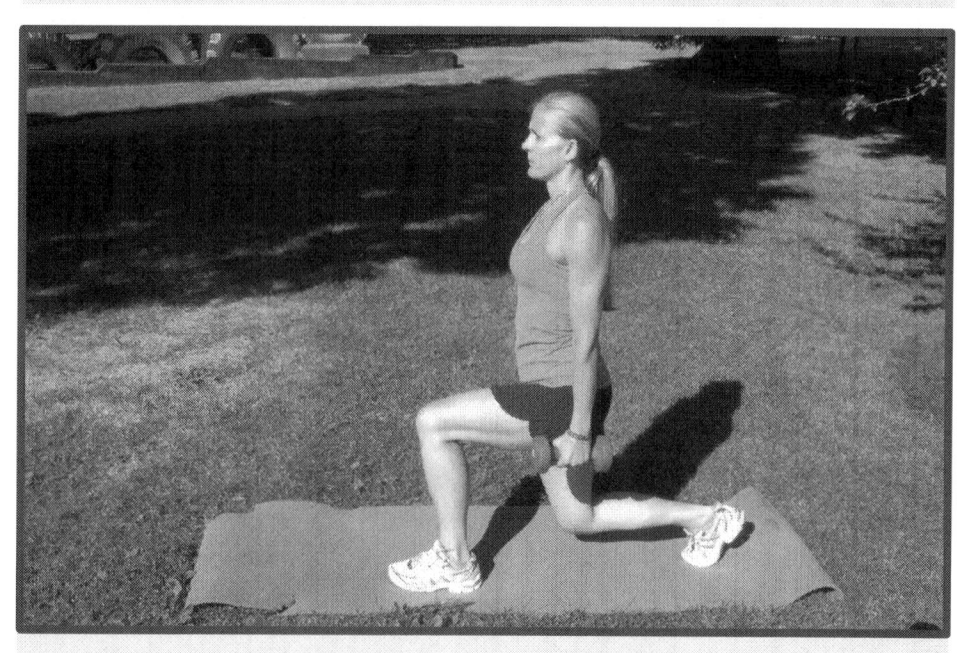

3. Kneel down so that your front knee is above your front ankle and front thigh is parallel to the ground. Look straight ahead and keep your back straight.

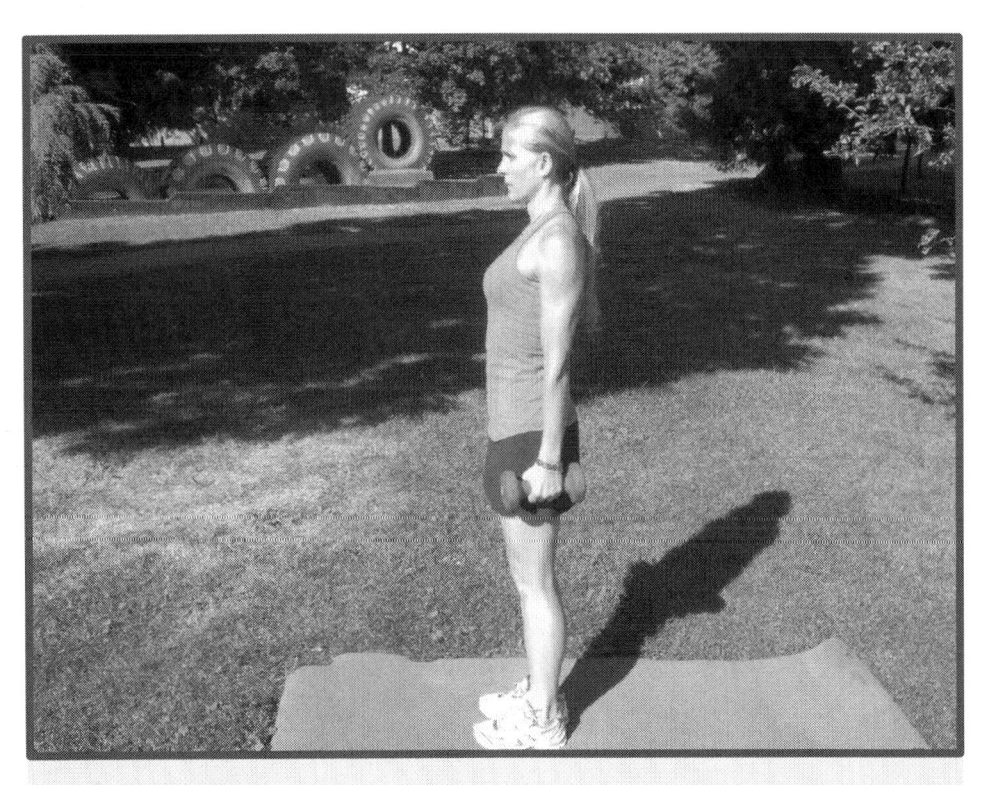

4. Return to the starting position with your feet shoulder-width apart and step back with your alternate foot.

5. Repeat 5-10 times each leg. Work up to three sets of 10-15 each leg before increasing the weight.

OVERHEAD DUMBBELL PRESS

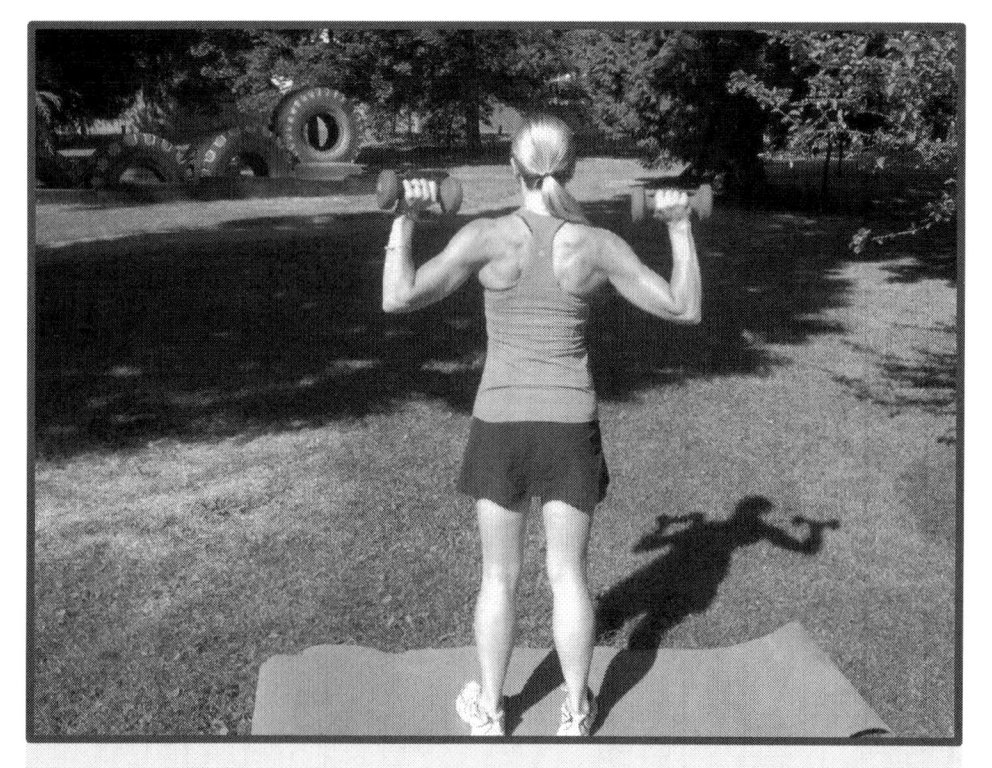

1. Stand with your feet shoulder-width apart. Hold the dumbbells so that your hands are facing upward and your upper arms are parallel to the ground.

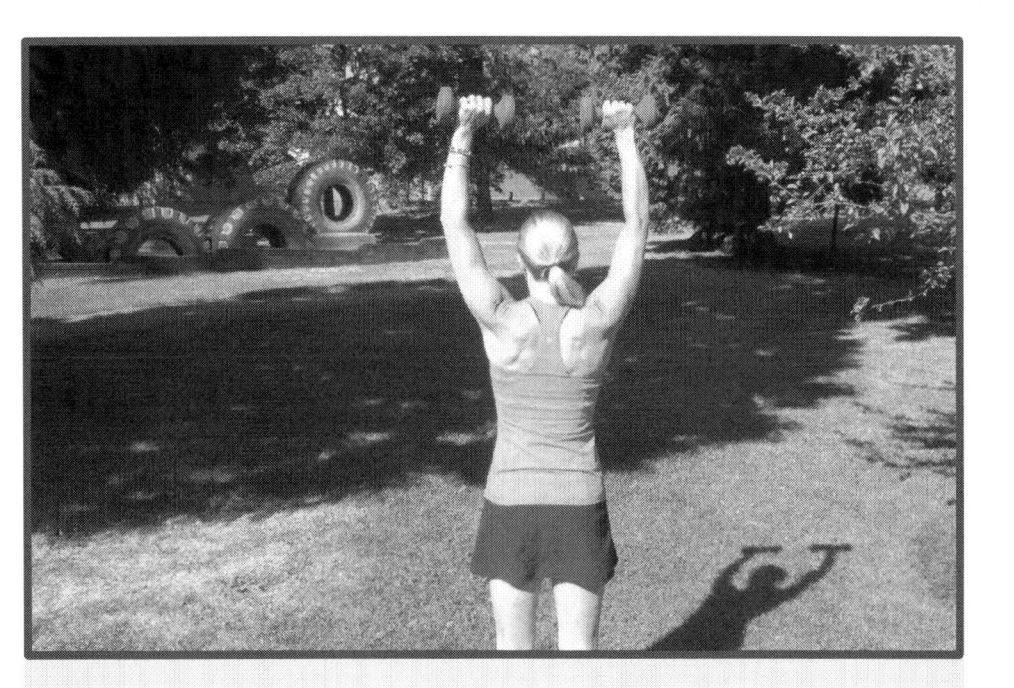

2. Press the dumbbells overhead in a smooth motion -of about two seconds-.

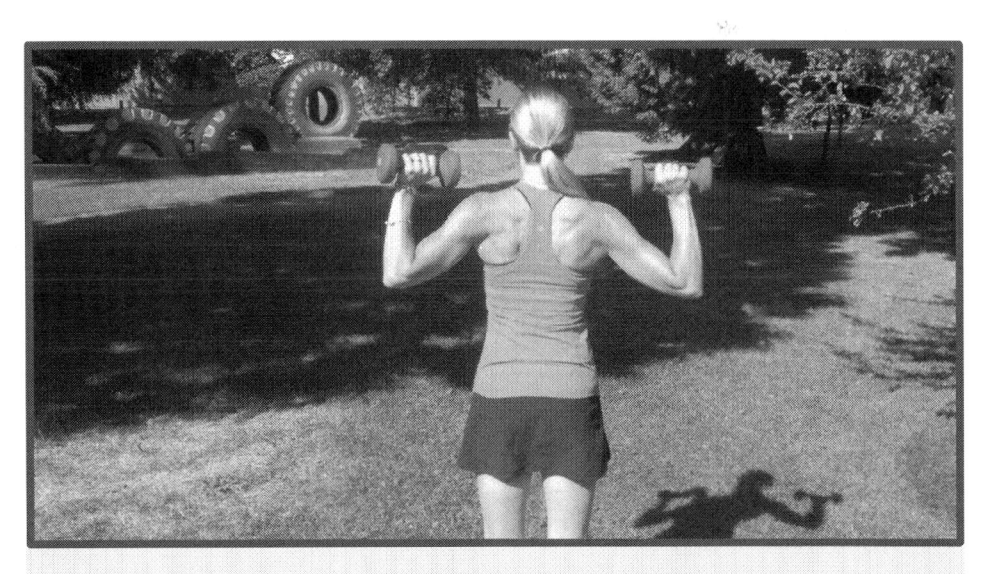

3. Return to the starting position and repeat for 10-15 repetitions.

BENT-OVER ROWING

You must keep a straight, flat back for this exercise.

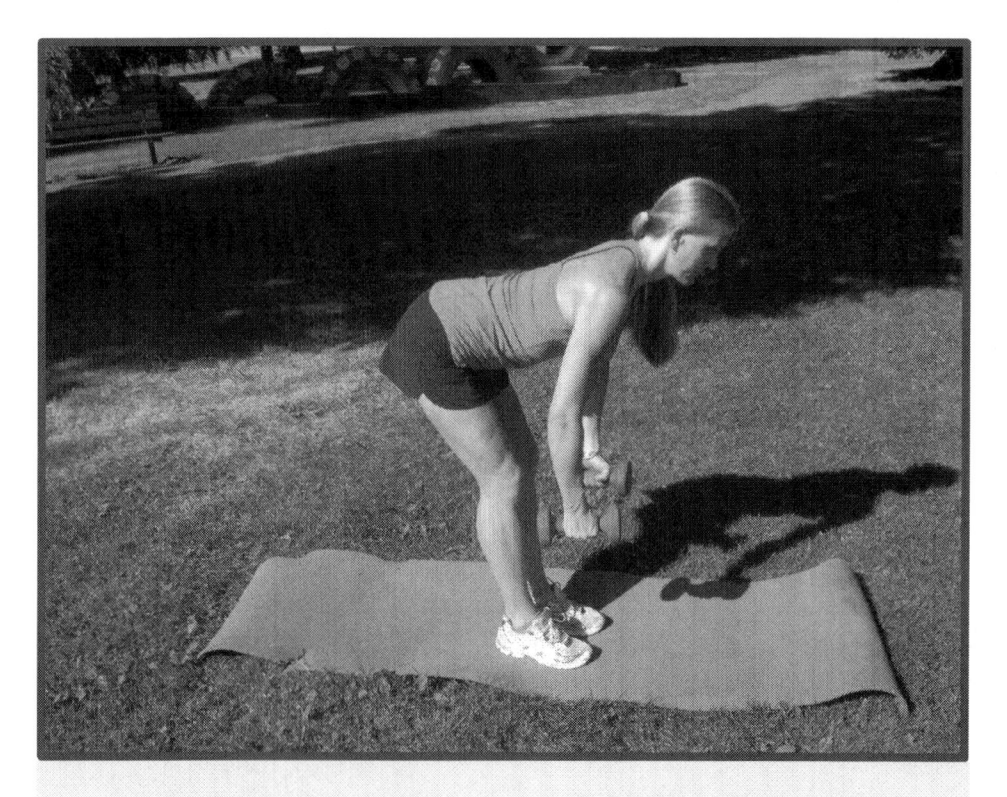

1. With knees slightly bent, bend over approx. 90° so that your back is parallel to the ground. Extend your arms with the weights toward the ground. Keep a slight flex in your elbows.

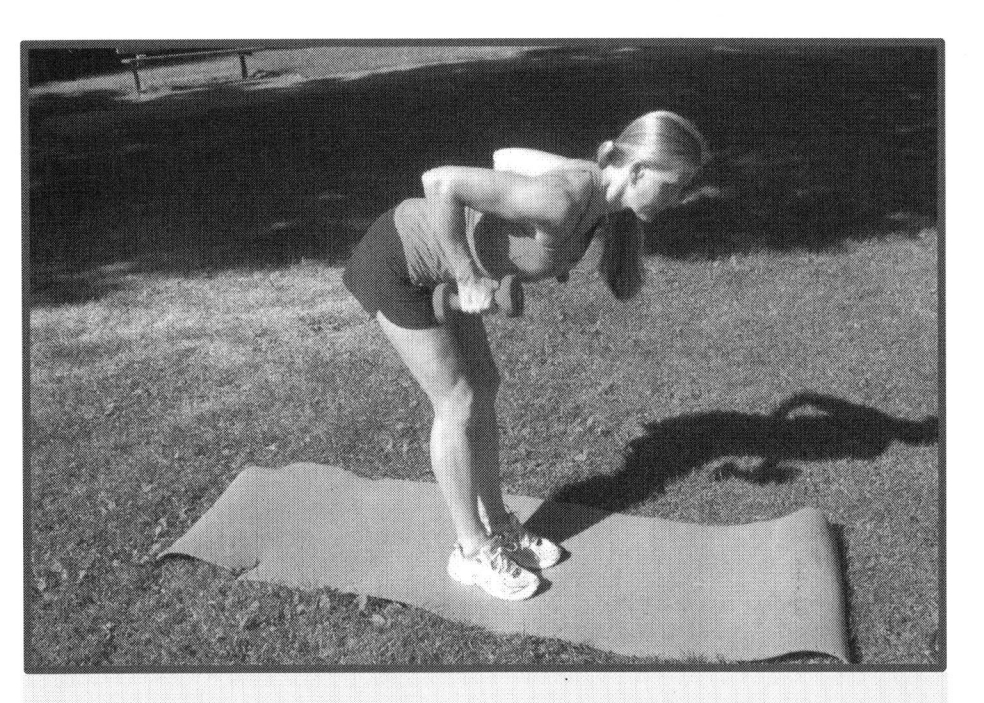

2. As you pull the weights toward your waist, squeeze your shoulder blades together.

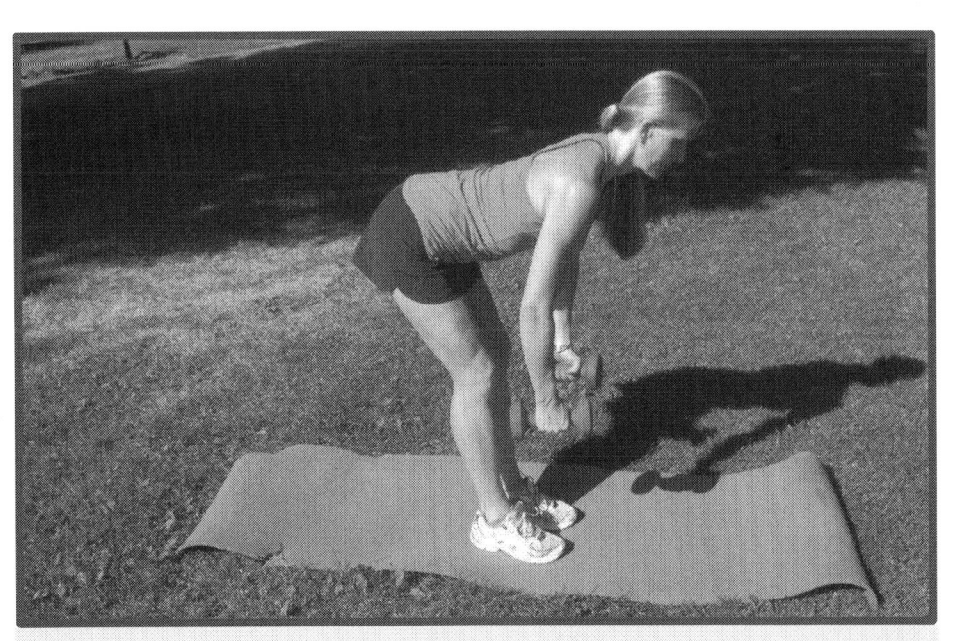

3. Extend your arms back toward the ground/floor. Repeat 10-15 times in good form. Do not swing the weights toward you. Work up to three sets before adding weight.

ROWING VARIATION WITH RUBBER CABLES

You can perform most dumbbell arm exercises with rubber cables/bands. The cables are cheap, light, easy to store and basically harmless if you drop one.

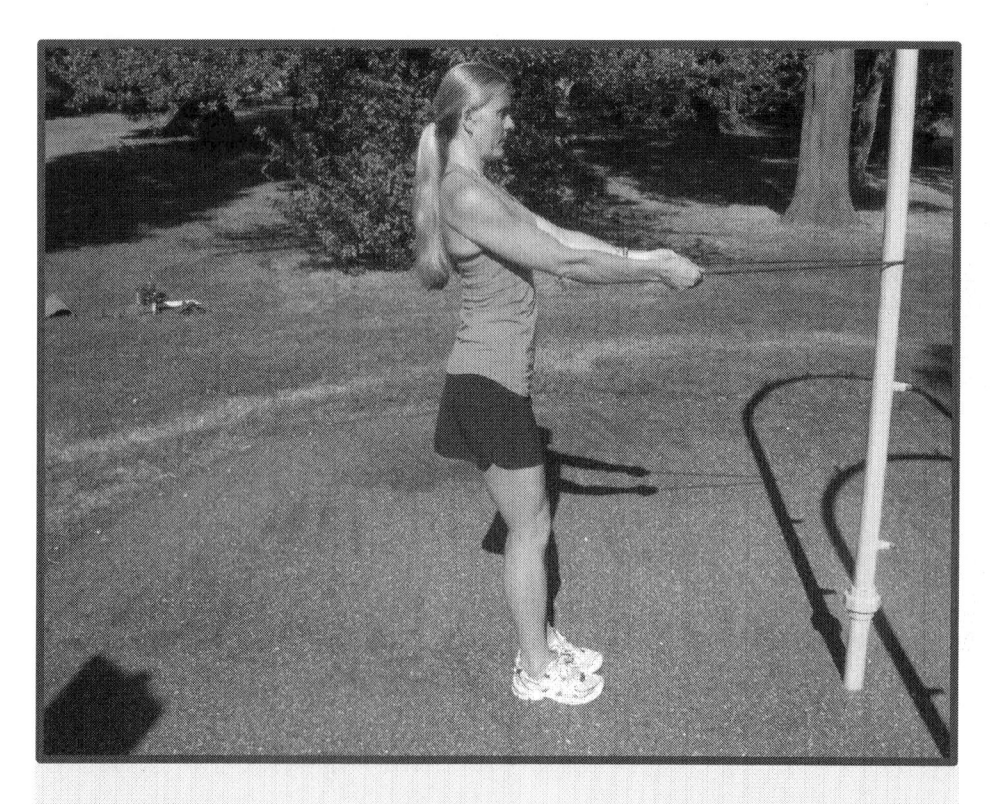

1. Keeping a straight posture and back, hold the ends of the anchored rubber cable with your arms extended. -You can anchor the cables on a fixed object, such as a pole, doorknob, or fence post. Just beware that it doesn't slip off and hit you.-

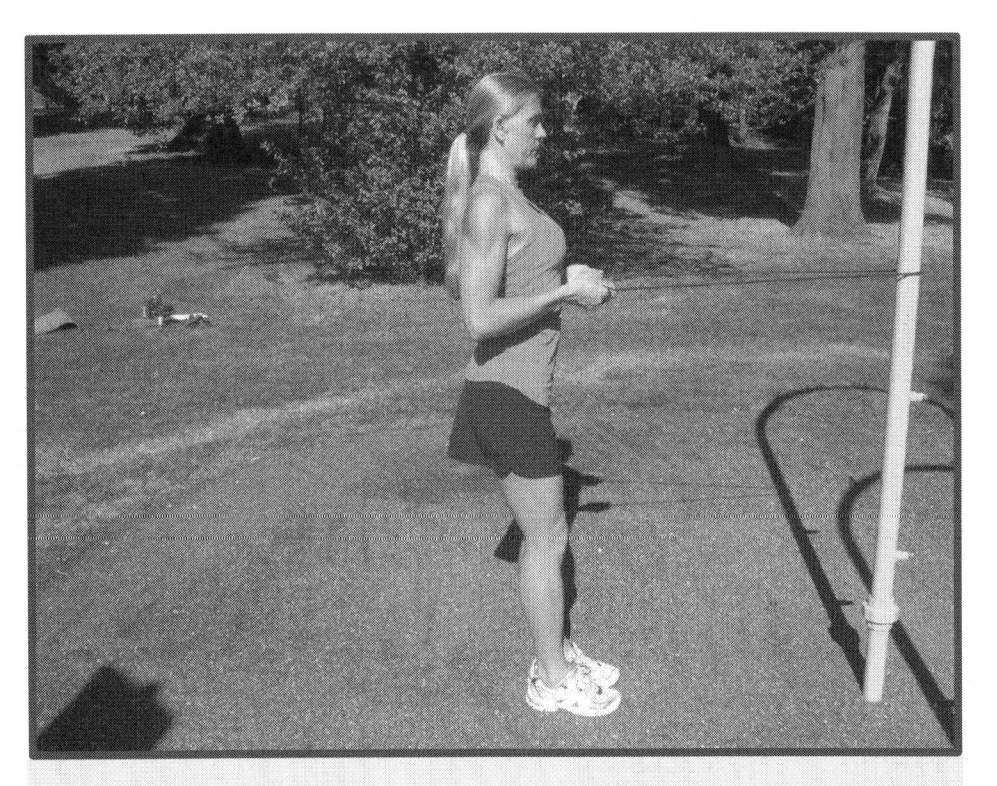

2. Keep your elbows in close and pull your hands to your sides, by your lower rib cage. Squeeze your shoulder blades together. Extend your arms, and repeat for 10-15 repetitions. One to three sets.

BICEP CURLS

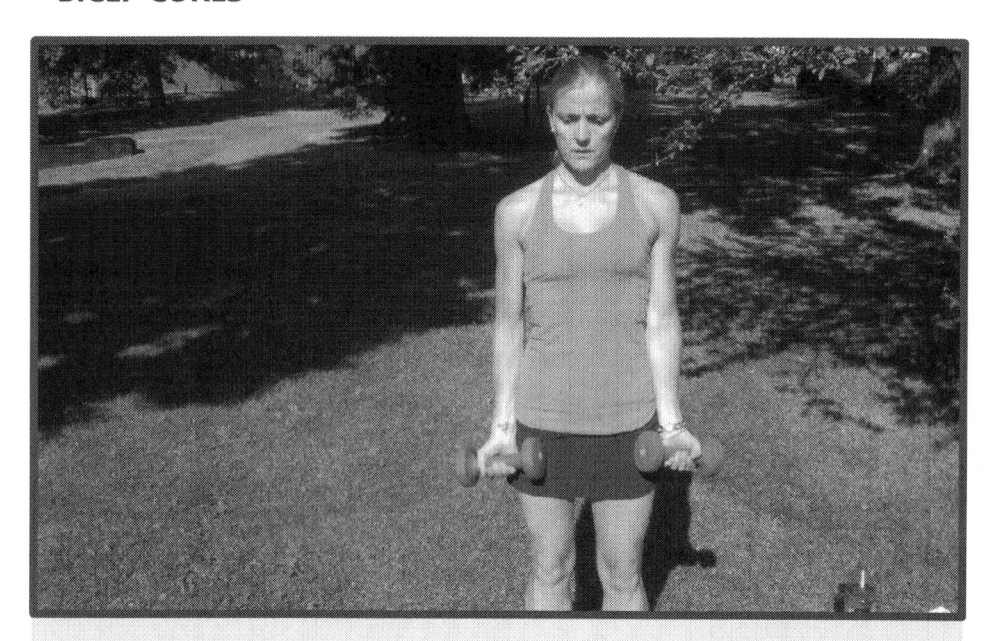

1. Stand with your feet shoulder-width apart. Hold the dumbbells down toward the ground with your palms facing forward.

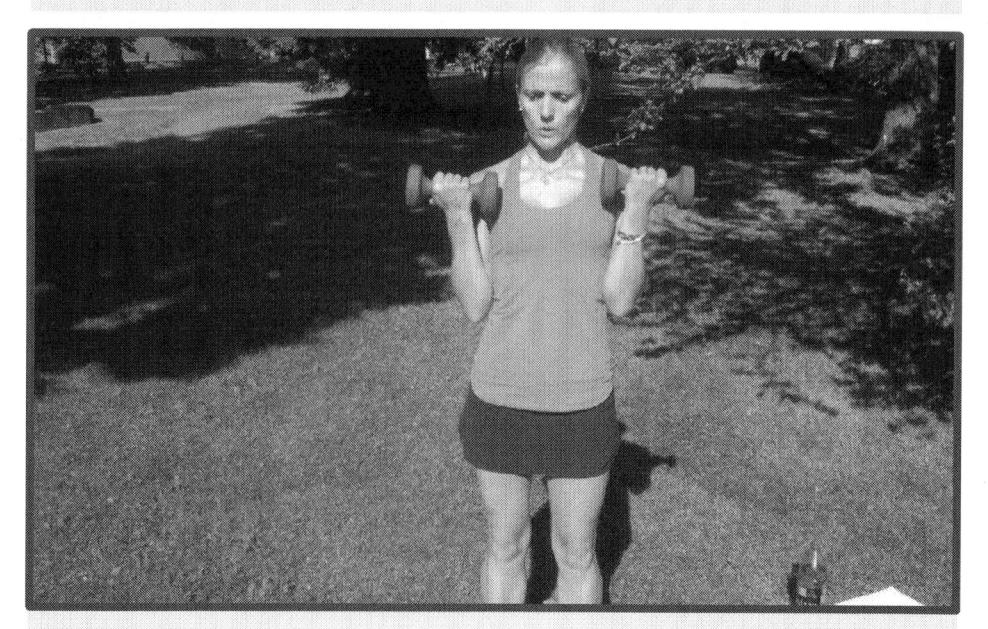

2. Keeping your back straight, raise the dumbbells toward your shoulders.
3. Pause, and then lower the weights. Do 10-15 repetitions. One to three sets.

BODY-WEIGHT EXERCISES -BWES

When I did not have access to a weight room, I started using body-weight exercises. Many exercises, from dancing, martial arts and sports to yoga and Pilates, are BWEs. I have found two simple yet effective BWEs are Hindu squats and Hindu push-ups. These exercises really demand the deep breathing you need to keep going strong. They also leave you with an "oxygen high" instead of the usual fatigue and muscle pain associated with most strength training.

HINDU SQUATS

If you are unfit or have knee problems, you can start out with half squats. I first read about Hindu squats -batiks- when I was a teenager back in the 1970s. It was a popular exercise for the wrestlers of India, who had phenomenal wrestling ability, strength and endurance.

See the steps to perform Hindu squats below.

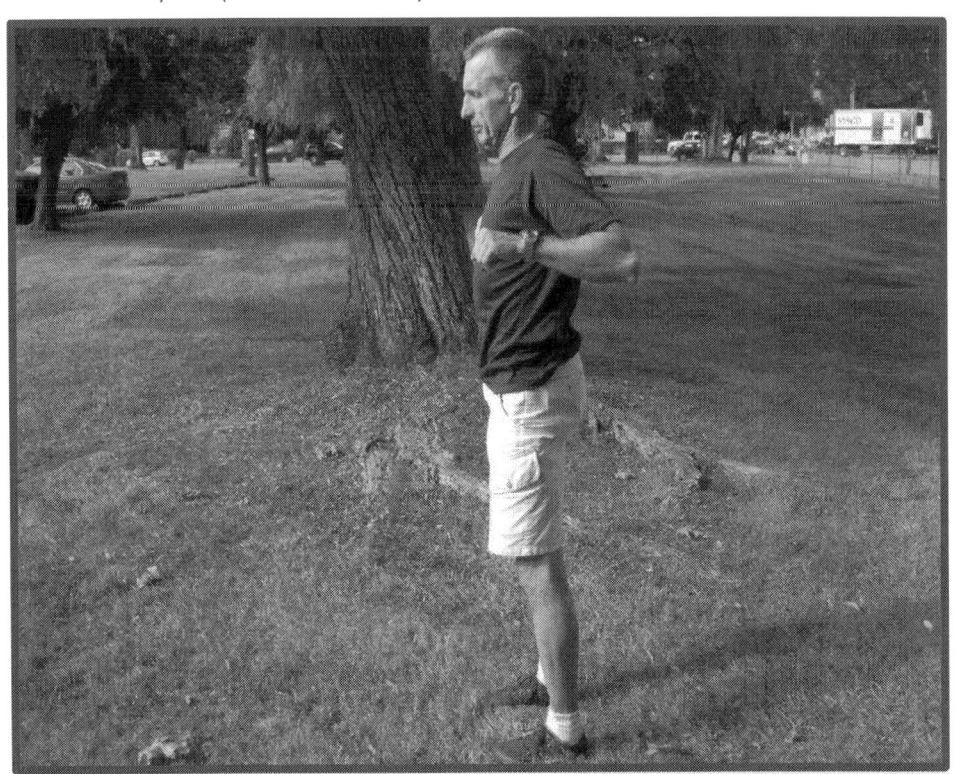

1. Stand with feet shoulder-width apart and your forearms held level with the middle of your chest, and elbows forced back so your wrists are near your armpits.

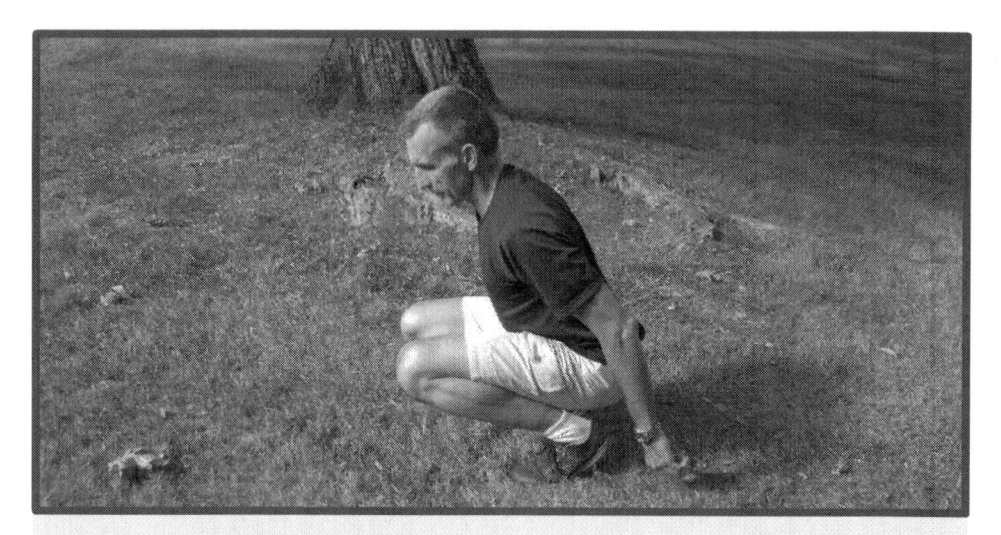

2. Keeping your back straight and your head up, bring your hands straight down and behind your back for balance. At the bottom of the squat, raise your heels and balance on the balls of your feet. Keep your body upright and your arms down. -Exhale.-

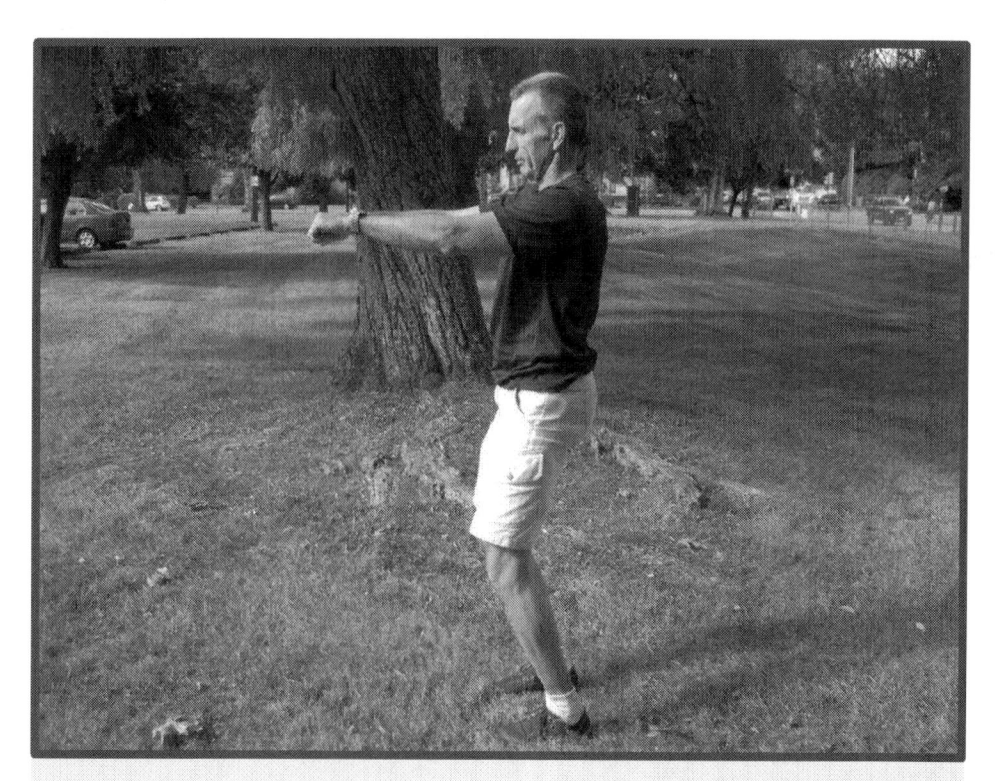

3. As you rise up, swing your arms forward at chest level, push off with your toes, and straighten your body.

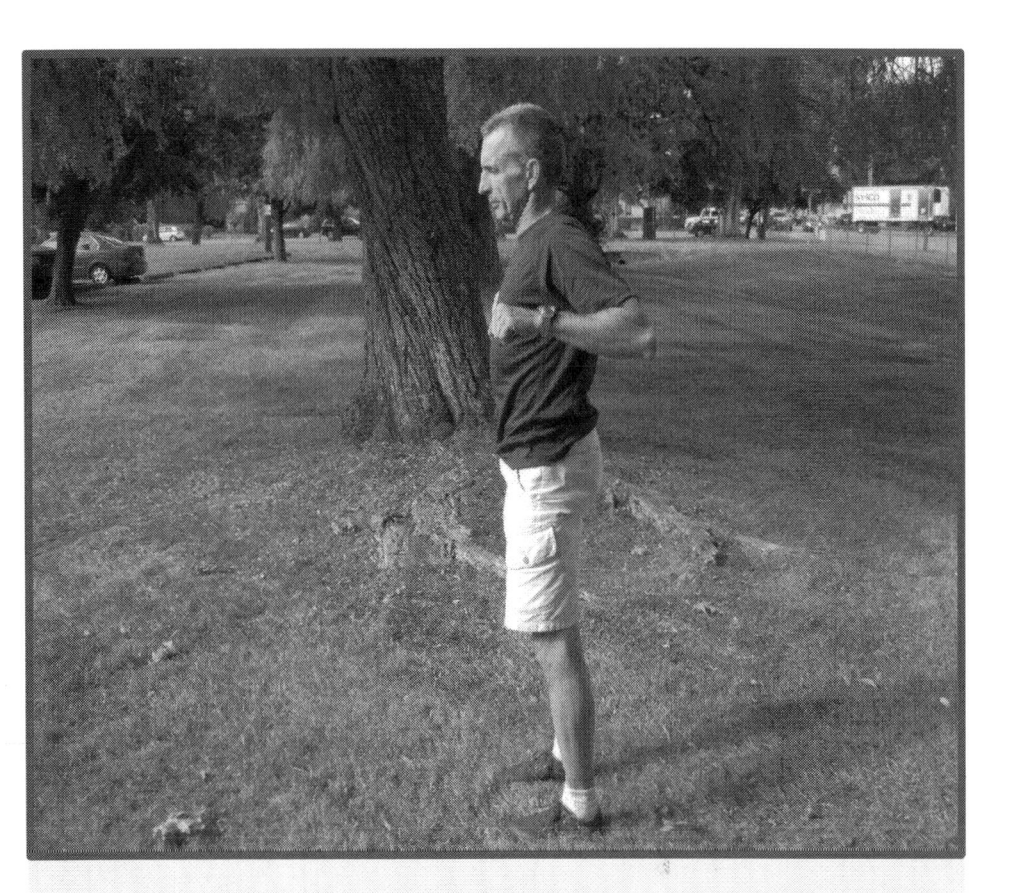

4. As you reach the height of the squat with your arms held forward at chest level, pull your hands in and your elbows back, and inhale.

5. Repeat

The breathing is the reverse of what you would do when squatting with weights. Instead of holding your breath -or inhaling according to some coaches and textbooks- on the way down and exhaling on the way up, you exhale on the way down and inhale on the way up.

When you get the hang of this exercise, go faster while keeping good technique. Again, you want to breathe out forcefully and inhale deeply.

This completely contradicts the mainstream -Western- knowledge of how to breathe when you exercise. However, if you have read the chapter on breathing and how some animals breathe when they run, you may be able to see the sheer genius behind this breathing technique.

When you squat down, your lungs, midsection and rib cage compress. As you stand, your lungs, midsection and rib cage expand. This is much like the running rabbit or dog that inhales as their forelegs and rear legs extend and then exhale as their forelegs and rear legs come together. As they run with a bellows-like action, their lungs force air in and out. The rabbit or dog's body does not fight itself to breathe while running.

HINDU PUSH-UPS

Hindu push-ups also operate in a similar fashion to the Hindu squats. As your head goes down, you exhale as your abdominal muscles, midsection, chest and lungs are contracting. As your head goes up, your midsection, chest and lungs are expanding. They are similar to the first portion of "dive bomber" push-ups.

The steps to perform Hindu push-ups are below.

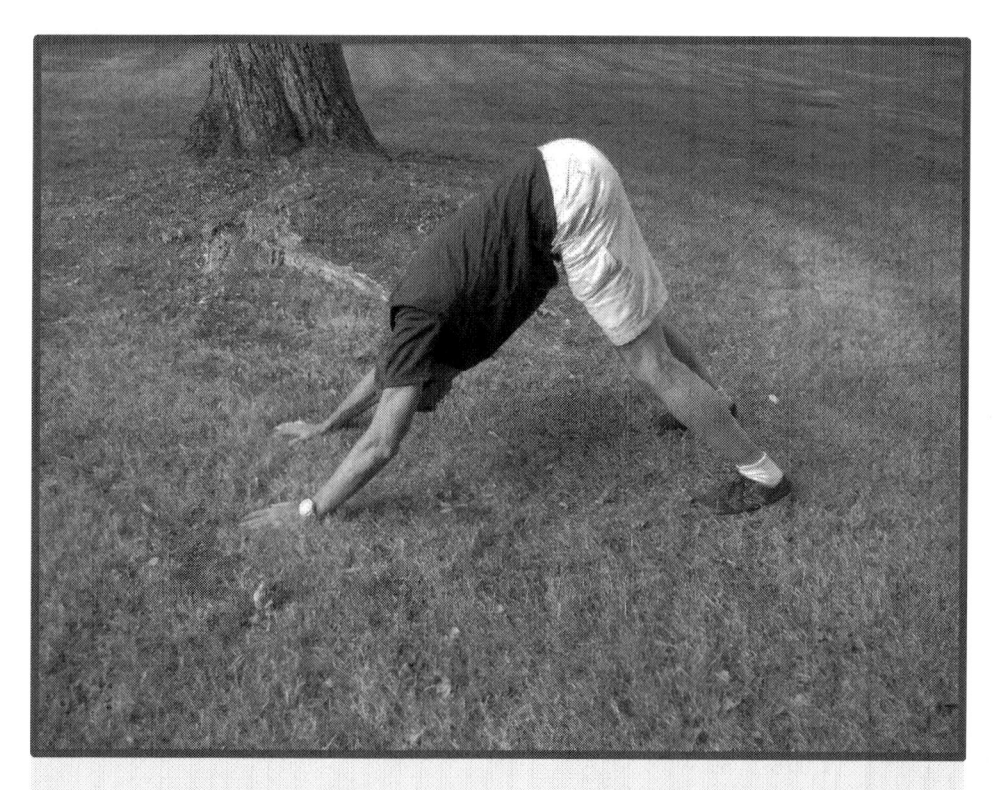

1. Start with legs wide and butt up in the air, like a wide-legged, downward dog yoga posture. Your arms are extended in front of you, about shoulder-width apart, and your head is downward, facing between your feet. -Exhale.-

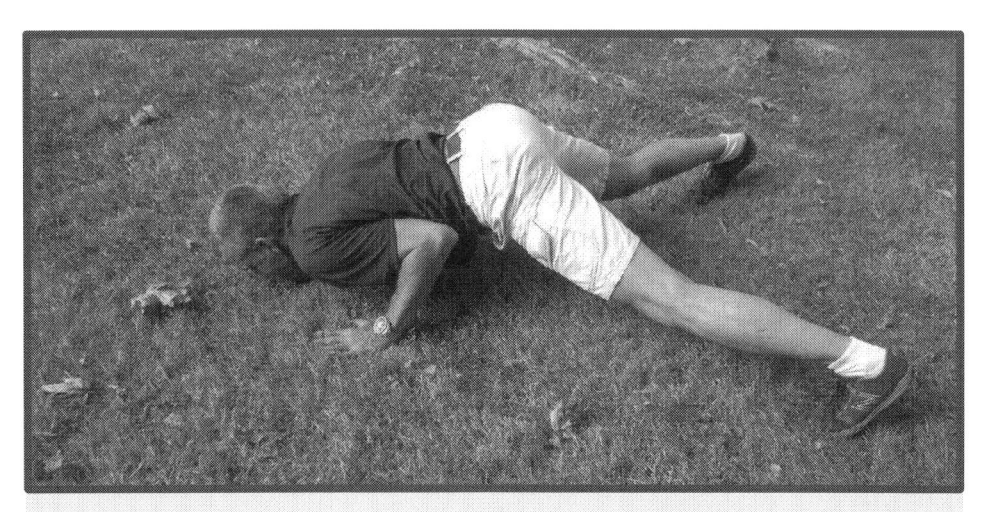

2. Bend your arms like a push-up and dip forward, bringing your nose, then chest, then hips close to the ground.

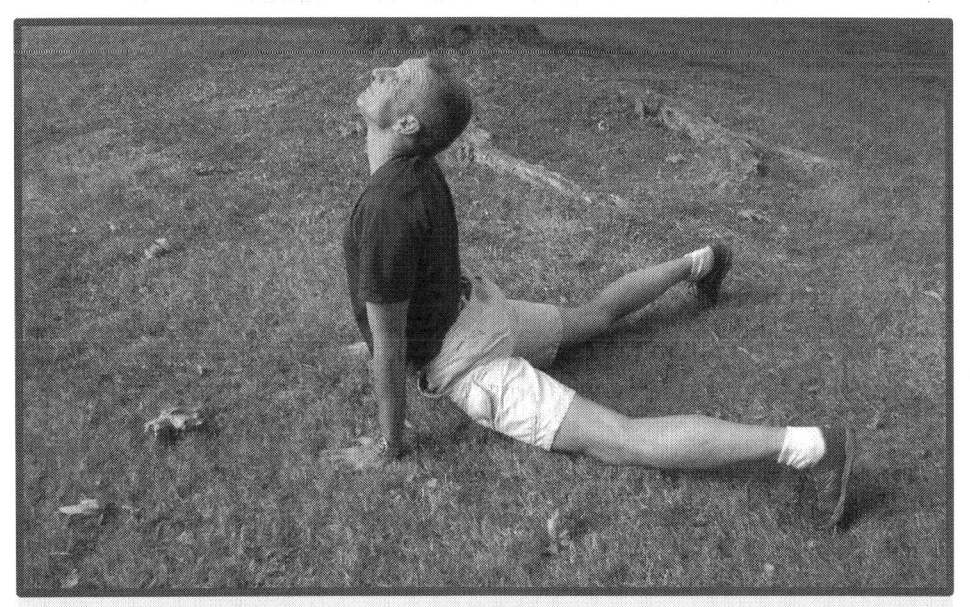

3. End with your hips almost touching the ground, your back arched and your head looking upward. -Inhale.-

2. Repeat

For a couple of months, I performed wind sprints in the sand, and two or three times a week, I did the Hindu squats and Hindu push-ups. After getting up to two sets of 100 Hindu squats and 60 Hindu push-ups, I was able to hike to the top of Mt. Rainier -14,000 feet- without too much difficulty -even as a youngster of forty-seven years old-.

Hindu squats gave me the lungs and leg power to get up to those higher altitudes that heavy squats or running would not have given me. And I doubt I would have had the same performance had I just been jogging or running long distance.

Full-range motions are extremely useful in grappling, martial arts, hiking and lifting things, such as children. -Bending over stiff-legged is a sure way to strain your back.- If you cannot squat down and get close to an object, it is difficult to lift it. While carrying heavy packs in the army, I was forced to frequently crouch with 25-50 pounds -11-22.5 kg- on my back. While core and leg strength was essential, the ability to stand up from a crouch or squat position was a handy asset. More so, it is freedom.

RETRO-RUNNING

I once asked a pretty Chinese lady, whom I saw walking backward in the evening in the Granville Island area, what she was doing. She explained that it was an exercise to reverse ageing. Since then, I have seen other older Chinese people doing the same.

This was pretty cool, as I have been retro-running -running backward- for several years to improve my footwork and stamina. I never realized there might be a health benefit to it.

Next time you are out for a short run, try running a few meters backward. At first, it may be a bit awkward and you feel like you are falling backward. Eventually, by glancing over your shoulder while you run, you will feel more balanced and aware of where you are going. After you get the hang of it, try changing forward, sideways, backward and forward again. You might be surprised how your speed improves.

Running backward or retro-running is initially about four to eight times harder than running forward -retro-running about a quarter of a mile is equivalent to running two miles-.

Runner Kat Clewley completed a full 42 km -26.2 mile- marathon backward in Hamilton, Canada. Boxer Gene Tunney regularly ran four to eight miles backward.[xiii] In 1927, Tunney defeated Jack Dempsey for a heavy-weight championship title. Another very famous backward runner was Bill Robinson[xiv] who officially ran 100 yards backward in 13.8 seconds. That is faster than most people can run forward. Bill "Bo Jangles" Robinson was known for his ability to tap dance and dance backward up staircases. He also taught tap dancing and starred with young actress, Shirley Temple.[xv]

I have found that running backward makes me much lighter on my feet. This helped me immensely later in life when I took up dance lessons. I adapted fairly quickly without looking too clumsy. Incidentally, ballroom and Latin dancing can supplement your training by making your movements more fluid. Dancing can improve your social life and take you into your later years with grace and coordination, while running and strength-endurance training can still leave you looking like a klutz on the dance floor.

FIRST CONTACT: FOOT STRENGTH AND HEALTH

For training purposes, I usually make a point of running barefoot whenever I can, especially on the beach, in the sand or in an area with grass. Running on the sand or grass teaches your feet how to absorb the impact as you run.

If you run on small gravel or pavement while barefoot, you learn in an awful hurry that the usual heel-toe method of running does not work. You learn really quickly how to run like most children or barefoot athletes run: on the edges and balls of the feet. Also, your bare feet will get massaged and various reflexology points will become activated as you run. The reflexology points will stimulate various organs of the body and improve your overall health. Try it and feel the difference.

Too much padding in running shoes has made many runners' bodies weaker, as there is a tendency to over-rely on the padding rather than proper foot placement. However, running on pavement for long distances requires either adequate padding or well-conditioned feet. I made the mistake of running a half marathon on pavement with my thin-soled trail runners. Even though I finished under a respectable 1:39:00, my lower back paid for it.

So, for good running technique and for feeling better overall, practice running barefoot -or even use trail runners on trails- when you can. Get the right foot protection for those long, hard surface runs.

TIME TO TRAIN

When I hear people complain that they don't "have the time," I am reminded of some top athletes who are very busy people:

- Kate Middleton is a tennis player and once lead a women's rowing team.
- Sheryl Crowe was a state champion hurdle runner who now plays tennis.
- Geena Davis was a competitive archer, placing 24th out of 300 women trying for the Olympics.

To find time, make the time. Cut out the unnecessary parts of your life, such as surfing the net and watching television, and you will be amazed at how much free time you really have.

RECREATION

Exercise is not all work and goal setting. The fun half of exercise is the recreational part. Walking, hiking, bicycling, swimming, sailing and various sports make activities more social and enjoyable.

Being past the fifty-year mark doesn't mean that you cannot enjoy the outdoors or activities at a local community center. One of my former personal training clients was a competitive badminton player at age seventy. The famous actor Abe Vigoda, who at age fifty-three played Detective Phil Fish on the sitcom Barney Miller, jogged regularly and played handball.
-When he showed up to audition for Barney Miller, he had just run five miles without time to shower and change. His tired appearance helped him land him the role that he played for seven seasons. Another example of how your fitness can pay off.-

IRIS DAVIS 76-YEAR-OLD BODYBUILDING CHAMPION

She holds the world record for twenty-one pull-ups at seventy-six years old and is an eleven-time National Physique Committee -NPC- winner. In 2020, Iris Davis was presented with the Pioneer award by the Women's World Leadership Congress.

Yet, the fitness champion had her share of obstacles to overcome. Born into a poor family in Dublin, Ireland, she had little thought of achievement. "Back then, women did not go to college," she recalled. Undaunted, she began to study on her own, even while working in a factory at age fourteen.

It was in the US that Iris made her humble start in weight training. It began in the early sixties when women were almost unheard of or not even allowed into gyms. At the time, Iris had suffered the loss of both her first child and her husband, leaving her a struggling widow. "In order to save my own life, I just started walking up and down a street," she comments. "One day, I walked into a gym and started working out.

"I couldn't believe how good I felt and copied all of the men's exercises. I have kept going for all of these years because I found that when I was in the gym, it was impossible for me to feel sad or depressed. And I've kept at it for fifty-four years. I wouldn't change the lifestyle for anything."

After successes in fitness and bodybuilding competitions, Ms. Davis began turning her attention to training others. Her clients range from young body builders to eighty-year-olds.

"I take delight in meeting people and telling them about health and fitness, especially since there are no women my age and generation who can now influence youngsters.

"I liked the way that I looked back then, and I set out to instinctively prove to myself that I could stay fit until I was fifty years old. Now that I am seventy-six, I realize that fifty is still a baby.

"I was never exercising for anyone else. I was doing it for myself. My advice to others is to do it for yourself. Keep fit and keep happy. And don't let anybody bring you down."

SUMMARY

Exercise for fun. Train for a goal.

Resistance/strength training trains your body to rebuild itself, increases bone density and burns fat more effectively than cardio exercises only.
- Retro-running and walking backward can improve your balance and endurance.
- Dancing can improve your balance and coordination.
- Make time to exercise.
- Exercise to feel good about yourself.

CHAPTER 07

PAIN, WHO NEEDS IT?

PAIN, WHO NEEDS IT?

"Just because you are in pain, doesn't mean you can be a pain." - Jasmine Mah, RMT

Pain takes much of the fun out of living. You know the crabby people who are in pain and constantly talk about their pain and make sure that you know about their pain.

Aside from injuries and serious medical conditions, you will find three basic sources of pain:

1. Dehydration
2. Muscle imbalance
3. Inflammation

DEHYDRATION

Dehydration can creep up on anyone, especially physically active people. I have seen soldiers and construction workers collapse from dehydration. Often people overheat and forget to drink water. Or, they overdress and overheat. This often happens in hot AND cold weather conditions.

A little-known fact about the cold weather is that IT SHUTS DOWN THE BODY'S THIRST MECHANISM. This is something that I had to pound into my own head and the people I had been training for arctic conditions. The body simply stops feeling thirst in the cold. Therefore, when in the cold, you must ensure that you drink enough water throughout the day. If you notice that your urine is bright yellow, you might be dehydrated and not know it.

You may have been working physically hard or exercising hard at the gym and wondered why you had a muscle cramp or a headache. The frequent answer is dehydration.

Even an office worker who has been sitting all day and drinking coffee may experience dehydration. This is often because the coffee is a diuretic and is drying out the drinker.

I came from the old army school of thought where we rationed our water or demonstrated discipline and toughness by denying ourselves water. Well, after several dizzy spells and muscle cramps, I have changed my philosophy. Drink when thirsty. But not to the point of being water-logged or when electrolytes are over diluted -hyponatremia-. Overdrinking water can be as dangerous and deadly as dehydration.

When water fails to quench your thirst, you might be running low on electrolytes. In that case, drink a mixture of water with a bit of salt. Over the years, I have used a simple solution of the juice of a lemon, a liter -quart- of water, a teaspoon of salt and a tablespoon of honey for replacing electrolytes. Even the Roman legionnaires used to drink a solution of vinegar or old wine to quench their thirst.

Forget about pop, coffee or alcohol if you are dehydrated. These items will draw water out of your body instead of rehydrating it.

MUSCLE IMBALANCE

If you are sitting most of your day, you are often going to experience rounded shoulders, a tight and weak lower back, tight hamstrings and tight hip flexors. Overly tight hip flexors can affect your lower and upper back, digestion and knees. Just look in any office and you will usually see people slouched at their desks with their heads leaning forward. To avoid this body warping, you need to stretch and stand up periodically throughout your day.

Many professionals take frequent breaks from their desks to move or do exercise. For example, writer Dan Brown -author of The Da Vinci Code- takes a break every hour to perform push-ups and sit-ups. Western writer Louis L'Amour used to punch a heavy punching bag during breaks. I find that a short walk or some stretches are enough to clear my head and release some tension when I have been at my desk too long.

Even if you exercise regularly, you can experience pain from muscle imbalances. A prime example is overemphasizing chest exercises, such as the bench press, and ignoring the upper back and back of the shoulders. This is what causes some weightlifters to have their arms rotate inwards with their knuckles facing forward, giving them a gorilla-like posture.

Another muscle imbalance example is too many abdominal exercises. All of the sit-ups in the world will not necessarily give you a flat tummy. After months of sit-ups and leg raises, I had developed a strong midsection with a big knot of muscles around my abdominal area. While it was great for taking hits in kickboxing, it gave the appearance of a muscular pot belly. Couple that with a slouching posture and I looked in poor physical shape. Later, when I trained in classical Chinese kung fu, my body became stronger and more aligned and my health improved.

Well-rounded exercise systems, such as dancing, classical martial arts, power yoga and Pilates, can remove and reduce pain in your body. As mentioned earlier, I noticed a relief in my former chronic hip and back pain after taking my Pilates instructor's course in 2002.

Many of my students also reported pain reduction after taking my Stomach Flattening or Pilates classes. One of my students, a provincial-level bodybuilder, reduced his chiropractor visits from twelve times to once per month. It was a simple matter of strengthening and stretching the right muscles groups.

You will find some useful exercises in Chapter 3, Posture, Power and -less- Pain. And visit www.2ndwindbodyscience.com.

INFLAMMATION

Inflammation often comes from stress in the body. The three biggest inflammation villains tend to be stress, food allergies and tooth decay.

STRESS

Excess stress causes the release of cortisol in the body. As the cortisol attempts to protect the body, it can cause inflammation, and movement becomes painful. Exercise, fresh air and rest can often relieve the pain of stress.

When stressed, I recommend that you keep moving. It will often calm you down and allow your body to flush out the cortisol and toxic byproducts.

FOOD ALLERGIES

Food allergies are one of the biggest culprits in pain. I know that if I eat too much wheat, dairy or sugar, my joints will sometimes ache. This can even cause inflammation in the brain, which I have found to make my thinking somewhat foggy after too many pastries. Other culprits can be nuts, shellfish, seafood, potatoes, tomatoes and citrus fruits.

One fast way to confirm that you are allergic to a food is to check your heart rate before and after you eat a suspected allergen. If your resting pulse rises significantly, then you are probably allergic. Another method is to just stop eating the food for a week and see if you feel better.

What makes these foods difficult to give up is that you will often crave the very foods that you might be allergic to. It can be very similar to giving up cigarettes, coffee or alcohol. However, as your body becomes cleaner, you will tend to reject foods that you used to crave.

So, reevaluate everything that you have been eating all of your life and note what might be the dietary culprit. Here is the watch list:

- Dairy: milk, ice cream, milkshakes, yogurt, cheese, pizza
- Wheat: pizza, beer, pastries, bread, gravies, most processed food
- Sugar: pastries, candy, chocolates, pop, processed breakfast cereals
- Shellfish: crab, oysters, clams, shrimp, lobster
- Alcohol: beer, wine, liquor
- Eggs: egg dishes, some baked goods

Keep in mind that when you are in good health, stress-free and in a good state of mind, you can feel next to indestructible and eat almost anything. In my bulletproof twenties, I worked out all of the time and consumed large amounts of beer, pizza and other items that were poor quality food. -But, hey, no one can tell you different when you are young, right?-

But it is still in your best interest to minimize the substances that are working against your health and fitness quest. If you really miss those foods, save them for a once-a-week cheat day.

Otherwise, here is the game plan to cut back on the allergic reactions that can cause drowsiness, allergies, mood swings, joint pain and the dreaded bloating:

1. Each week, cut out a suspected offending food, such as milk, eggs, shellfish, sugar or wheat, for at least five days and observe how you feel.
2. Observe what happens after a day of NOT eating a hyperallergenic food. Note the possible withdrawal symptoms, such as cravings, runny nose, and foul taste in your mouth.
3. After five days of not eating an allergenic food, try to reintroduce it and watch what happens.
4. Take your resting pulse prior to consuming the allergenic food and

observe whether or not your heart rate increases or any other reaction.

5. Note which foods you keep making excuses to eat. -Mine are ice cream, yogurt, dark chocolate and red wine, thank you very much.-
6. When you do eat an allergenic food, do not beat yourself up over it. Just take note and minimize the amount that you eat. Also note when you tend to eat these foods.
7. Watch out for those times that you were stressed, rushed or feeling "hangry." Think about when you were most vulnerable, such as Hungry, Angry, Lonely and/or Tired -HALT-.

This can be a difficult quest, as many people have grown to like the allergy buzz or comforting numbness. That is normal. Remember, it took years -or decades- to build a tolerance and reliance on the allergenic foods. And it might take a few weeks to clear it up and years of vigilance afterward. But trust me-it is worth the effort.

Supplements that have been proven to build allergy resistance are

- Vitamin C: 500 mg three times per day. Avoid time-release formulas, as your body may treat it like an invader in different parts of your intestine.
- Vitamin B5 pantothenic acid: 1500 mg per day
- Vitamin B3 -niacin-: 100-500 mg. Start out in low dosages, otherwise you may experience about fifteen minutes of a flushing reaction that is scary to some people and uncomfortable. If you experience this flush, drink plenty of water.
- Probiotics

TOOTH DECAY

Even the ancient Greeks recognized how removing a decayed tooth could relieve a person's joint pain. I can speak from the experience of having to take painkillers for weeks while waiting for a dental appointment. Fortunately, the root canal work solved the toothache and joint ache problems.

Of course, there is still the possibility of tooth decay even with completed root canal work. Here is where the science of oil pulling might be able to help. Oil pulling has been used for thousands of years in Ayurvedic medicine. Basically, you swish around a tablespoon of vegetable oil in your mouth for twenty minutes, then spit it out and brush your teeth. Coconut oil is the best, as it contains antibacterial and antiviral properties. The twenty minutes goes by quickly while you are doing chores, working on the computer, or exercising.

Now, the first time that I did this, I almost threw up as I spit out some nasty stuff into the toilet. But over the next week, I noticed some improvement in my joint pain and had brighter, whiter teeth. Even if you are still skeptical, give it a try for five days and note the difference.

HERBS AND SUPPLEMENTS FOR JOINT PAIN

GINGER

One of the simplest and cheapest cures for joint pain can be ginger tea. Just chop up an inch of a ginger, simmer it in a pot of boiling water or a cup and drink throughout the day. I have read about and heard about pain relief results from both scientific papers and friends who regularly drank fresh ginger tea.

TURMERIC MIX

Turmeric tea and spice also work for joint pain. However, this is the most potent formula that I have used:

Tumeric, ground	1 tsp
Ginger, ground	1 tsp
Cardamon	¼ tsp
Cinnamon	¼ tsp

Put the mixture in a tea bag and steep in hot water for three minutes. Drink one to three cups throughout the day. These herbs are great for lessening joint pain, calming the stomach and even lessening depression -in some people-.

SERRAPEPTASE

Serrapeptase is a proteolytic -protein-dissolving- enzyme found in silk cocoons. Some sources are made from bacterial cultures. I have had good, long-lasting results using this supplement, especially when training infantry soldiers out in the middle of the prairies while I was still in my fifties.

A couple of my friends also swear by serrapeptase. One had recovered from a bomb blast in Afghanistan and now works up in northern Canada keeping bears away from worksites. The other sustained many injuries from boxing, bull riding, nightclub bouncing, military parachuting and a plane crash. If it works for these guys, it might be your ticket to less pain. Serrapeptase is available online and in most health food stores.

GLUCOSAMINE, CHONDROITIN SUFATE, and MSM

I have had mixed results with glucosamine, chondroitin sulfate and methylsulfonylmethane -MSM-. Chondroitin sulfate also claims to build up the joint tissue as does the MSM. The active ingredient in the last two supplements is sulfur, which is also important for clear complexion, skin, nails and hair. Sulfur is also found in the insulin hormone to regulate blood sugar. It is abundant in meats, fish and legumes.

Some studies report that some people feel better after taking these supplements. Yet, some people also felt worse and demonstrated signs of glaucoma, blood thinning and allergic reactions.[xvii] It is your choice to try them•or not.

CHAPTER 08

NATURE'S LOAN SHARK

NATURE'S LOAN SHARK

Would you expect top performance from your cell phone if you only recharged it about to 10% each day? Probably not. The same might be said for your mind and body, if you run them hard day after day without recharging.

Yet we do it all the time. Day in, day out, skipping rest and staying up late at night fretting over the day or watching mindless television.

Sometimes in real life, we have to push our limits and go without rest and sleep. I know in the army, I was required to miss rest and sleep for days at a time. And my deepest respect goes to the mothers of the world who run on very little sleep caring for their babies and children.

There are a few high-performing people who function well on very little sleep. But I found out -the hard way- that I function better with good, sound sleep. This has served me well in kickboxing competition, while serving in the infantry and with the -Canadian Airborne Regt.- paratroopers as well as in university. and just day-to-day living.

Experienced athletes and performers usually seem almost docile before a competition. They relax and conserve their energy for their event. They rarely run around all stressed out before stepping onto the playing field, mat or stage. Some do, but many do not.

Unfortunately, there is this misconception that missing sleep will burn fat. This is totally false as the lack of sleep will cause the body to bloat. This is often evident in some late-shift workers who miss sleep, such as some police, nurses and paramedics.

Lack of sleep can cause the following:

- Excessive cortisol
- Digestive disorders
- Elevated stress
- Lack of Human Growth Hormone -HGH-
- Depression
- Lack of concentration
- Stress and more stress
- Mood swings
- Predisposition toward diabetes

HOW TO GET A GOOD NIGHT'S SLEEP

- Get a good, firm mattress. Do the best that you can within your budget. But remember that most people spend several times more on their automobile than their bed. They might only drive the automobile a few hours per day, yet they spend six to eight hours a day on their bed. Something to think about.

- Strive for a dark bedroom. Get the heavy curtains or blinds. I noticed a much deeper sleep when I installed heavy curtains in my bedroom. They shut out both the light and most of the outside noise.

- Avoid heavy meals, caffeine, alcohol or violent movies just prior to going to bed. These stimulants will tend to keep you awake. Some people are conditioned to late-night eating and some alcohol before going to sleep. These people often skip breakfast in the morning and appear to function well otherwise. Find what works for you.

- Take 200-500 mg of the amino acid tryptophan -usually sold as L-tryptophan-. Ingesting tryptophan an hour prior to bedtime usually brings on a deep sleep. It is nonaddictive, and I have been using it occasionally for decades. You can also get your dose of tryptophan from turkey, chicken, fish, peanuts, eggs, cheese and sesame seeds. I have gone from getting up two or three times a night to visit the washroom to sleeping through the entire night just from winding down, darkening the bedroom and taking 300 mg of tryptophan.

Get your sleep. You owe it to yourself. Good sleep will not only improve your physical health, but it may prevent you from going into depression, which you will learn about in the next chapter.

CHAPTER 09

BRAIN BOOST

BRAIN BOOST

"You have power over your mind-not outside events. Realize this, and you will find strength." - Marcus Aurelius

Ever forget someone's name? Then you wait around, hoping that someone else will use their name or you have a chance to discreetly ask a friend who that person is.

I have been in this situation a few times. Sometimes, I wondered if my mind was going or I was not very attentive in the first place. And after a couple of concussions, I became really concerned about losing my memory, concentration and cognitive abilities, especially after watching people who I always thought were smarter and more intelligent than me decline in their mental abilities. Fortunately, there are methods to improve our abilities to think and remember.

YOU ARE SMARTER THAN YOU THINK

When I turned thirty-nine, friends encouraged me to toward higher learning, which enabled me to progress from a C-average high school student to a university graduate, instructor and author. Fortunately, you can do the same.

I have spent decades with soldiers, coworkers and trainees who constantly berate themselves for being stupid. And on occasion, I have also played this game. Being ignorant or "not-so-smart" is a safe place to be. Maybe your peers, a teacher or some other adult told you as a child that you were not too bright. After a while, you might've played it safe and accepted the status quo. I know this because I bought into this safe place where you do not have to think very hard and not much is expected of you. It kind of lets you off of the hook when something goes wrong. "I am just a_____-fill in the blank-. So, I can't be held responsible."

To start with, most people have brilliance in certain areas of their lives. For instance, I have a dyslexic friend who is a very good martial artist and painter. Singer and actor Cher has both dyslexia and dyscalculia -cannot make sense of numbers-. I have trained soldiers who had difficulty learning simple movements and skills but could assemble equipment after a brief glance.
Or the soldier who seemed so slow to learn and then quickly adapted to the outdoors like a wild animal. People can amaze you with their abilities, once given a chance.

And I am always amazed at how many women can carry on conversations and multitask at the same time. Multitasking, in itself, is the sign of a highly organized mind.

Consider the eight different intelligences: logical-mathematical, linguistic -languages-, musical, spatial -ability to envision three dimensions-, bodily-kinesthetic, intrapersonal -self-knowledge-, interpersonal -social skills- and naturalistic -knowledge of nature-. The people who may be slow in some areas, for example logical-mathematical intelligence, can be brilliant in other areas, such as languages.

You probably know people who can barely balance a check book yet are brilliant in sports, social interactions or even music. You can also recognize the many things that you can do that other people struggle with-not to mention the massive amounts of organizing, managing, calculating, communicating and physical tasks that you do each week.

So first and foremost, to become more intelligent, you have to recognize your current intelligence and ability to learn more. You would never have gotten this far without being able to think, plan, remember, negotiate and work. Give yourself some credit.

PRACTICAL WAYS TO IMPROVE YOUR MIND
TAMING THE STRESS BEAST

Few things kill brain cells or cloud the mind as well as stress. In fact, a single socially stressful event can physically destroy brain neurons.

One example is from back in 1996 when I found myself in a confused state, wandering up and down Osborne Street in Winnipeg, Canada. The accumulation of stress, at that time, had me confused on what to have for lunch. Finally, I settled on soup and a sandwich. It was a very strange feeling that I refuse to repeat.

You might have had a series of stressful incidents while attending high school or college. Sometimes personal stressors, such as money problems, can inhibit your ability to learn. I found that taking fewer courses enabled me to have more time to study and improve my marks. Another strategy is to budget ahead of time so that money problems do not interfere with your studies.

The other stress reducers have been mentioned already. In case you forgot, they are exercise, nutrition and rest.

LEARNING FASTER

Many of us were taught in school by book smart people. Not people smart. Book smart. They have this amazing ability to memorize whatever they read or hear. Then they think that the rest of the world learns like them.

But we also learn by discussing, telling stories, visually drawing, assembling or physically performing and practicing a skill. Take history, for example. It is far easier for me to learn about history through historical fiction and visuals than brute-force memory work from a textbook. So, to remember a fact, you can make up a story in your mind. When I taught subjects for the military, I often added a story or humor to maintain the trainee's interest.

Turning words into pictures often assists me with memorizing places and names. For example, someone's last name might be Hankins. So, you can think of "Hang Kings" and picture a king being hanged. It also helps to repeat the person's name three times to yourself and even envision it on their forehead.

Even when memorizing sequences, you can form pictures and stories in your mind. This can be applied to a list of several items, for example cup, dictionary, desk, ball, rock, kettlebell. You can imagine a cup with a dictionary inside of it. The dictionary is then slammed down on a desk, which is balanced on a ball and a rock. The rock has a handle and is used as a kettlebell.

ACTIVE MIND

There is good news about the human brain. At one time, it was believed that brain cells never regenerated and were considered permanently gone if damaged. The good news is that the brain can learn and adapt through neuroplasticity. The more that you use your brain, the more neuron connections are grown. So, keep your brain active. This means reading more instead of watching television and listening to audiobooks instead of your car radio. Even taking just fifteen minutes a day to learn something new will improve your ability to remember and understand.

Remember Chapter 1 on reprogramming your mindset? Being able to link an activity, for example learning, with something enjoyable makes that activity easier to perform. So, if you enjoy your subject and your class, memorization comes easier.

If not, I have used the same method for writing and sometimes exercising. Namely, I give myself small rewards for studying a textbook chapter or writing a page. After a while, your mind looks forward to studying in order to accept the reward in the end.

MUSIC

Music helps the brain study. I use something fast-paced when I am doing repetitive work that needs energy and not much thought. However, for study and writing, I prefer something more easy listening. -Thank you, Barry White and Shirley Bassey.-

EXERCISE

You already know the many benefits of exercise. Exercise increases oxygen and nutrients to your brain as well as releasing feel-good endorphins.

I like to exercise first thing in the morning, followed by a high-protein, complex-carb breakfast, such as eggs and oatmeal and minimal sugar. This gives me the alertness I need to work and write for several hours.

During your day, you should move around and go outside for at least a few minutes throughout the day. The sunlight and fresh air tend to trigger your mind to be more alert.

SUMMARY

- You are smarter than you think.
- Stress can inhibit your thinking and destroy brain cells.
- You can learn faster through continual effort.
- Keep your mind active, not just mildly entertained.
- Music can stimulate memory and concentration.
- Exercise releases stress and stimulates the brain.

CHAPTER 10

DETOXING THE BODY, MIND AND SPIRIT

DETOXING THE BODY, MIND AND SPIRIT

"The simple truth is that we are living in a sea of toxins and it is destroying our bodies and brains." - DR. HYMAN

Just the phrase "They went into detox" conjures up visions of drug-saturated celebrities and athletes who were sent away to some exotic place to recover from years of overindulgence. These places give rise to images of where the wealthy elite are counseled, massaged and fed in peaceful settings away from the hurried outside world.

Or so they say.

Detoxing or the classic cleansing can be as simple as short or long fasting, diet changes, herbal supplements, saunas and a bit of solitude. It is really not that painful, scary or complicated. In fact, I have performed my own detoxing or cleansing without even thinking about it. It was sometimes known as "too busy to eat" or "nothing left in the cupboards." Often, these bland diets of oatmeal, vegetables and beansprouts actually kept me healthy during economic lean times.

Anyone who has ever done home renovations or even just painted a room quickly realizes the importance of getting rid of the old building materials. Detoxifying does the same thing. It is meant to remove excess undigested matter from the intestines. This can include allergens, parasites, yeast and heavy metals. You can be eating the best food in the world but may still feel sluggish if your intestines are backed up with various undigested junk.

Just think about how one's internal plumbing gets plugged up in the first place.

Many people in the civilized world gobble down pounds and pounds of highly processed and difficult to digest "foods." Hamburgers and French fries are prime examples. The processed beef on a white flour bun and the deep-fried potato starch fried in old oil is hard enough to digest without the sugary soda pop that goes with it. This fast food is often eaten on the run. So, the hastily eaten meal is usually not chewed thoroughly before being washed down with some kind of fluid. This means the partially chewed
food does not get completely digested, assimilated or absorbed. Worse yet, the undigested mass can stay in the intestines too long and ferment. This fermentation forms hostile bacteria, gas and irritants.

Now, if you are able to eat a fresh tasty meal, say a chicken salad, in a pleasant surrounding with good company, I would say that the digestion process will be much more effective. This is why I admire lunch hour in parts of Europe, such as Germany, where people enjoy two-hour-long lunch

One-Day Cleanse	Eat fresh salads and steamed vegetables. No dressing.
Three-Day Cleanse	

On the first day, follow the One-Day Cleanse. Second and third days

Breakfast	Plain oatmeal or a vegetable smoothie
Lunch	Vegetable soup and salad
Supper	Baked root vegetables and brown rice

On the fourth day, gradually add protein foods.

Breakfast	Oatmeal with butter and cinnamon and/or vegetable smoothie
Lunch	Salmon salad, soup
Supper	Roast chicken and vegetables

breaks. There is plenty of time to enjoy your meal and have plenty of energy to work the rest of the day.

If your diet has been looking a little too much like the typical North American diet from Chapter 5, here is where a simple cleanse can help your body clean itself out:

It is interesting that many cultures celebrate religious holidays with fasting and prayer whereas many others in the civilized world tend to gorge themselves during these holiday times.

CLEANSING THE BODY

In addition to the simple cleansing diet above, introduce one or all of the following in order to further cleanse and detoxify your body.

SAUNAS

I recall regularly visiting a steam room right after instructing my Sunday night fitness class. Those nights, I always seemed to sleep the soundest.

Whether the sauna is wet, dry or infrared, it will help rid the body of toxins, raise infection-fighting T cells and relax the muscles. It is a small wonder that so many cultures value their steam rooms and hot baths.

COLON THERAPY

I had just spent two nights on the cold ground out in Shilo in Manitoba, Canada, then went to The Herbal Infusion Health clinic in Winnipeg. I was feeling physically beat from the weekend of training with the army reserves. But I had agreed to at least try a colonic irrigation. I really did not like the idea of a tube going up you-know-where. Yet there was evidence of the benefits of this procedure. So I gritted my teeth and proceeded to get irrigated.

Well, after getting flushed and flushed•and flushed out, I finally went to the toilet. There, I proceeded to have six -count •em- heavy movements as it were. Even though I was physically fit at forty-one years old, I could not believe how much waste that I had been carrying around. That night, I had one of the deepest sleeps that I can remember. When I woke the following day, I felt mentally alert and very clearheaded.

The experience made me think about how about many people must be worse off than I was with bloated colons and backed-up intestines. Since then, I visit the colon therapist about once a year or so and always feel better afterward.

CLEANSING HERBS

My favorite liver cleansing herb is milk thistle. It is cheap and available at most health food stores. There are many others, but milk thistle is simple to take and has few side effects.

CLEANSING THE MIND

When I was away from home with the military, I often did not see a newspaper or television for months at a time. And for the most part, I didn't miss them at all. When something was really important, like maybe the rise in gas prices, a sports event or a war breaking out, someone would pass it on through word-of-mouth. The same thing happened when I went traveling through Europe or Asia. I found that my mind was less cluttered during those times.

But once back in the city with school and civilian work, I became overwhelmed again with media, commentaries, advertisements, flyers, newspapers, memos, television and radio. Consequently, I often felt kind of hurried and had difficulty focusing.

To mentally cleanse, you need to give yourself some quiet time during the day and during the week. It might be as simple as reading a book in a quiet place, walking the dog, running on the beach, listening to calm music or meditating. At first, it may feel unproductive and pangs of guilt may override your efforts. But if you set aside that fifteen minutes or more of time, you should find that your mind calms down and jumps around less frequently.

When you can afford a whole weekend or two days off or more, you might like to go out of town to someplace different, to look at the sights and relax. If at home, you can go biking, hiking or walking around an unfamiliar area. Leave the cell phone, and bring a book or go with a friend. These mental cleanses or time-outs can improve the rest of your week.

CLEANSING THE SPIRIT

I might call this type of cleansing spiritual, as it gives a person a chance to reflect on what is really important to them. This should not be confused with escapism, where the urge is to "get away from everything," numb yourself and then reluctantly return to real life at the end of your trip.

The spirit cleanse is a retreat from the people, places and situations that wear on you. I found that working out of town during the summer gave my head a break from dealing with difficult customers, negative people and unsatisfying work. Often when I returned to work, I could see things through a fresh perspective and was less annoyed.

THE 24-HOUR BODY-MIND-SPIRIT DETOX

You can put together your own detox day during the week or weekend. One of my clients used to go to a spa with her friends or a short trip out of town.

If you do not have that luxury of extra time and money, you can do something as simple as eating a vegetarian supper the night before, retiring to bed early, skipping or having a light breakfast and going to a sauna -or hot yoga- and then having a lunch of fresh vegetables. The whole time, you can avoid television, radio, media and cheap gossip. The whole idea is to give your mind and body a chance to recharge.

SUMMARY

- Periodic cleansing diets can improve your digestion, immune system and body's recovery.
- You can cleanse your body with fasting, diet, saunas and colon therapy.
- Mentally cleanse yourself by avoiding unnecessary information.
- Cleanse your emotions and spirit by removing yourself from annoying situations.

CHAPTER 11

BEATING THE BLUES

BEATING THE BLUES

"I'm not grateful for depression, but it honestly made me work harder and gave me the drive that I have to succeed and make it work." - LILI REINHART

Have you ever known the feeling of lonely days, failure or a broken heart? Chances are, you probably have. At the very least, you find out what you are made of and who your friends are. But even mild depression is an unnecessary burden. So let's beat the blues before it tries to cramp your style. Let me show you the drug-free solutions that have worked for me and many others.

EXERCISE

"Hey," the voice from over 3,000 kilometers -2,000 miles- away said, "I heard what happened."

He was calling me from Southern California to one of the coldest cities in North America -Winnipeg, Canada-. I had guessed that my friend Rob was referring to my recent breakup and maybe my debts along with my failed real estate project. -He probably had no clue that my heat had been cut off and I was sleeping on an old army air mattress. You might say that the black dog of depression was scratching at my front door.

After we had talked for a while, he added, "Keep exercising. Just keep exercising."

Then and there, I made a pact with myself that until I was working full time and financially stable, I would:

1. Not consume any alcohol. -I was NOT going down that path to skid row.-
2. Get up early every day to work or look for work.
3. Eat three times a day.
4. Exercise every day.

And exercise, I did.

Even after a full day of work, I would practice martial arts forms in my basement, perform chin-ups on overhangs and do push-ups anywhere. Then I would run and run. Sometimes five, ten and even eighteen kilometers. I would exercise myself to fatigue and then sleep deeply.

For cheap food, I ate eggs, canned beans, oats and rice. I used cheap vitamins wherever I could find them. Some was better than none.

Most important, I changed my environment. I got out of the run-down neighborhood, with gang graffiti, break-ins, two murders and my slashed car tires. I teamed up with a friend and moved into a cheap but affordable apartment. I was able to get full-time work, design fitness workouts -Stomach Flattening and Cardio Kickboxing-, put in proposals to the city and rent space for instructing fitness classes.

Instructing fitness classes was the best thing that ever happened to me. It put me in front of positive, enthusiastic, high-performing people. The classes were more than income and fun. Teaching those classes gave me a sense of purpose and increased my circle of friends.

A year later, at age thirty-nine, I entered university to earn a Bachelor of Human Ecology. Even while attending university, I stayed physically active. I still taught fitness classes, worked with the army reserves, and ran three marathons. Physical activity always helped relief my stress, period.

You too can use exercise as your own natural Prozac.

NUTRITION

Look at the way many depressed people eat. They often really don't give a damn about nutrition and eat mostly highly processed, sugar-laden, white flour products. These depressed people are also often angry -as anger is usually a symptom of depression- and live on coffee, cigarettes and alcohol to fuel an already depleted set of adrenal glands.

A high-protein and slow-carb diet is as simple as the following:

Breakfast	Eggs and oatmeal
Lunch	Roast chicken and a salad
Supper	Salmon, steamed vegetables, brown rice

You can even adjust for when you eat fast food:

Breakfast	Egg muffin, scrambled eggs or oatmeal
Lunch	Chicken burger without the bun or two chicken wraps
Supper	Chinese stir fry but skip the white rice and sweet sauces

It makes you wonder whether their attitude gives them poor health habits or their poor health habits give them bad attitudes.

More than the psychologist's couch, you need a steady flow of energy from your food. As I mention several times, the high-protein, slow-carb type of eating will help maintain a stable, healthy blood sugar and energy levels.

People sensitive to blood sugar changes, like hypoglycemics, have much in common with depressed people and some alcoholics. In fact, 86% of Dr. Mathews-Larson's hypoglycemic patients reported feeling depressed.[xviii] Mathews-Larson put her patients on low-sugar and low-caffeine diets and reported that most of her patients experienced relief from depression. Even AA founder, Bill Wilson, found that by reducing caffeine and sugar in his diet, he felt better than just attending the group therapy meetings.

The other nutrient that most people are lacking -and afraid of- is fat. Yes, the dreaded three-lettered word. If you fear eating fat, you must learn the difference between good and bad fats, which is discussed in Chapter 5, Eating, Energy and Entertainment.

In his book 12 Rules for Life, Dr. Jordan Peterson stated that many patients were cured of anxiety just by getting regular sleep and eating a high-protein, high-fat breakfast in the morning.

SUPPLEMENTS

A sample of a daily healthy mind-body formula is as follows:

Multi-B vitamins	50 mg of each B vitamin, except 50 mcg for B12
Vitamin C	500 mg
Calcium-Magnesium 2:1	300 mg of calcium & 150 mg of magnesium
Fish oils	2 capsules -or 1 T of good quality cod-liver oil-
St. John's Wort [xx]	1-2 cups of hot water with 1 T of crushed herb; occasionally

To stabilize blood sugar, Dr. Mathews-Larson recommends niacin -vitamin B3- and chromium. About 500 mg of niacin with breakfast and at supper and 200 mcg -micrograms- will help stabilize most people with low blood sugar.

When I was a Morse code operator in 1978, I discovered the benefits of mega dosages of B vitamins. After taking them for two months, I felt better, drank less alcohol, felt calmer and decided that I wanted a better career than the one I had first chosen. B vitamins, like thiamine -B1-, help convert nutrients into energy, especially the brain and nervous system. Cobalamin -B12- is important for mental function and is mostly found in animal sources. B vitamins in general are very unstable and are often lost during storage, cooking and processing. Therefore, you might be deficient in multiple B vitamin supplementation.

I will also mention the value of calcium and magnesium for calming the nerves, muscle growth, and a healthy cardiovascular system. Deficiencies of magnesium have been linked to suicide.[xix]

Another proven supplement and nutrient are fish oils. As a child, I was given cod-liver oil during the wintertime. This was a good idea, as cod-liver oil is very high in vitamin D, which helps reduce depression. With our current lifestyles of indoor living, lack of sunshine and the fat scare, we have become a vitamin D-depleted society. Therefore, you need to get outside for a bare minimum of ten minutes of facial sunlight per day.

FRIENDLY BACTERIA

Aside from affecting digestive health, bacterial balance is also important for the neuro messages that travel from your gut to your brain. This is because the bacteria can affect your body's supply of serotonin. Serotonin, which influences mood, sleep, depression and aggression, is more concentrated in the gut than the brain. Something like 5%-10% is stored in the brain and the remaining 90%-95% is in your intestines. This might explain the problems of antidepressants raising serotonin in your brain and not your intestines. Even though the brain and intestines produce serotonin separately from each other, their nerve messengers will still affect each other.

A study at the University of Toronto School of Medicine and Department of Nutritional Sciences demonstrated the effects of beneficial bacteria on humans with Chronic Fatigue Syndrome -CFS-. Thirty-nine people with CFS were randomly given either twenty-four billion Colony Forming Units -CFU- of Lactobacillus casei -found in yogurt- strain Shirota -LcS- or a placebo over two months.

After two months, the people taking the LcS probiotics showed a marked decrease in anxiety, including better sleep, less dizziness and shortness of breath, and fewer appetite changes.

A similar study involving mice was reported in the December 2011 Journal of Neurogastroenterology and Motility. In this experiment the probiotic Bifidobacterium longum was found to reduce anxiety behavior in mice with colitis. Better bacteria meant happier mice.

There are a few things that you can do to get the benefits of brain-enhancing, fat-reducing intestinal flora:

- Reduce all white sugar. This means even artificial sweeteners. A 2008 study at Duke University found that rats fed Splenda had a significant reduction of good bacteria in their in their digestive tract.

- Eat fermented foods. They are good tasting and cheap. Many ethnic stores have kimchi, Japanese natto, East Indian dahi and sauerkraut much cheaper than the main supermarkets. Learn to make your own.

- Avoid sweeteners. This means eat only plain yogurt or kefir.

- Use probiotics. I find that the Greens-type of probiotics works well for me. -I have no commercial connection with any of the brand names mentioned.-

ENVIRONMENT

The other factor in keeping the black dog of depression at bay is your environment, as mentioned in Chapter 1, the mindset chapter. Changing your environment, including people, work, industries, location and time of day, can affect your mood and well-being.

When I moved to a better neighborhood, I slept better, enjoyed going home more often and experienced a stronger mental focus.

RUBY'S STORY

"My biggest roadblock in fitness has been depression," explains Ruby, a sixty-four-year-old retiree. "Being depressed is like falling into a rut in the road. It is a BIG rut. It is DARK. You feel like there is a weight on you. But on the other side of the thing holding you down is a weighted blanket. Kind of like a comfort place. Take a lazy person and times it by ten, and you get the idea.

"When I am in this state, I don't answer the phone or go anywhere for days."

Prior to her bouts of depression, the former army clerk had always been physically active. While serving in the Canadian Army, she ran and performed regular Physical Training -PT- every working day, regularly carried a 45 lb. -20 kg- rucksack, practiced shooting firearms, and worked outside in hot, cold and wet weather conditions. She prepares her own meals of fresh food and avoids milk, wheat, white rice, white salt and Canadian-made pasta. Instead, she prefers pasta made in Italy -Bosa brand-.

To stay physically fit, Ruby forces herself to get up at 6 a.m. and "get out the door" with her dog, a blue heeler, by 7 a.m. Together they cover 5-7 km six times a week. When building up to longer distances, Ruby follows the Jeff Galloway method of training. Namely, walk for a count of 100 and then run for a count of 200. She also trains using High-Intensity Interval Training -HIIT- during the week. "I like the way it makes me feel," the former sergeant explains. "I find yoga too slow. I need to feel like I worked out. It is important to find something that you like to do."

As for dealing with depression, Ruby works with an "intention circle" of kind people. "If you have good intentions, you will draw good things to you. If someone needs help, we have an intention circle. This is where we all focus for a few minutes on someone's problem with a positive outcome."

So far, it has had good results.

"Most important," she advises, "Try looking after yourself every day."

SUMMARY

Depression can be prevented or reduced through exercise, nutrition, supplements and environment changes.

To prevent or reduce depression you will

1. ____Do something active every day.
2. ____Increase protein and slow carbohydrates in your diet.
3. ____Take B vitamin and other essential supplements every day.
4. ____Spend a minimum six hours per day in a happy, energizing environment.
5. ____Get a good night's sleep.

CHAPTER 12

ROADBLOCKS, DETOURS AND OPEN HIGHWAYS

ROADBLOCKS, DETOURS AND OPEN HIGHWAYS

"When you come to a roadblock, take a detour." - MARY KAY ASH Now is the time to anticipate those speed bumps, hairpin curves and roadblocks that might have been programmed into your psyche and will often make their appearances.

This is perfectly normal. Whether it is starting a new business, running a charity or working on a six-pack of chiseled abdominals, there is a strange force that wants to drag most of us back to "normal" -whatever that is-. This force seems to want to drag us back to where we are comfortable and "put us in our place." In fact, it hates change. "It" just keeps coming back.

So, it is time to starve out the beast.

1. Strengthen your environments. Go to the places and people that inspire and uplift you. Remember, you can often influence where, when and who with you want to be. Use this choice.

2. Use routines and rituals. Rituals build success. When we talked about environments, we are also building rituals that program success. During martial arts training and the military, we followed rituals at the beginning and end of training. We also wore uniforms For better or worse, these rituals or routines reminded us of where and who we were and that we were about to learn or train.

3. Make it hard to "fall off the wagon." If you really want that chocolate éclair, cigarette, shot of rum, bad company, extra thirty minutes of sleeping in, late-night movie, etc. then you have to make yourself pay for it. Make rules.

    Yep. Do something uncomfortable. Scrub a toilet, do fifty push-ups, hold a half squat for five minutes or talk to the most obnoxious person that you know. I used to give myself one hundred push-ups if I wanted to phone a friend or surf the web instead of studying. Sometimes I would do the push-ups and then the violation. But usually, I became too tired to the point where that small voice in my head said, "Forget about it!"

4. Ignore perfectionism. This is a clever form of procrastination. Your mind will sometimes make excuses not to do something because the situation is not perfect. Too cold, too hot, not enough gym space, etc., etc.

5. Dump the toxic relationships. Toxic relationships can be family and so-called friends who make fun of your dreams and aspirations, coworkers -"that will never work"-, nasty clients/customers, low-end neighborhoods, an unsatisfying career, or overbearing spouses or partners.

   As mentioned in the first chapter, on mindset, the simple process of changing your environment can be a tremendous boost to your energy. Your environment can mean people, places or activities. I had a friend who progressively became more stressed, less healthy and verbally abusive over the course of thirty years. During the last couple of years, I always felt let down after visiting him, especially when he was in a wheelchair and in his final days in the hospital.

   At least two of my friends and clients dropped over fifty pounds very quickly after they broke up with their partners. You might know people like this and wonder what happened when they suddenly look better and start acting more outgoing. Quite often they did a bit of "relationship housecleaning."

   There was a pretty, kind of plump woman in one of my fitness classes. After I wrote up a high-protein diet for her, she dropped several pounds. Then she became a Pilates instructor and looked amazingly trim. About the same time, she dropped her boyfriend and her job and went on to start a new business. The boost to her fitness seemed have given her that "I can" attitude.

6. Have a training partner or group. This can work for or against you depending on the people you hang out with -see above-. Help each other out.

7. Keep track of your progress with a journal and graphs.

8. Above all, be good to yourself. Hey, look around. Look how far you have gotten, while others have fallen away, quit or are even not with us anymore. Celebrate your small victories. When you are kind to yourself, you are often more kind to other people.

······························

RESOURCES

JOIN US ON FACEBOOK
https://www.facebook.com/groups/1932464357068828

FREE HEALTH, FITNESS & CONFIDENCE-BOOSTING NEWSLETTER
www.2ndbodyscience.com

COACHING, CONSULTING, WORKSHOPS & TRAINING
https://www.2ndwindbodyscience.com/contact/

i. Amino acids are the building blocks of protein. Your body can manufacture about fourteen of the twenty-two amino acids. The other eight must come from food sources. Animal sources, such as beef, chicken, fish and eggs, are complete proteins whereas vegetarian sources are often incomplete and require intelligent combining to meet protein requirements.

ii. Romaniello, J. & Bornstein, A. -2013-. Man 2.0 Engineering the Alpha: A Real World Guide to an Unreal Life. HarperOne. P. 96

iii. Cadman, B. -2020-. How to remove cortisol from the body naturally. Medical News Today. Retrieved from https://www.medicalnewstoday.com/articles/322335#why-is-higher-cortisol-an-issue

iv. Macdonald, F. -2018-. This is where body fat actually goes when you lose weight. Science Alert. Retrieved from https://www.sciencealert.com/where-body-fat-ends-up-when-you-lose-weight

v. Collins, K. -2006-. Why the French don't get as much heart disease. NBC News. Retrieved from https://www.nbcnews.com/id/wbna11145653
The French generally eat less and are more active than North Americans.

vi. Kirschmann, J. D. & Dunne, L. J. -1984-. Nutrition Almanac. McGraw-Hill.

vii. Perricone, N. -2002-. The Perricone Prescription. Harper-Collins. Pp. 75-107.

viii. Pearson, D. & Shaw, S. -1983-. Life Extension: A Practical Scientific Approach. Warner Books, Inc. P. 111.

ix. Fredericks, C. -1988-. Psycho-Nutrition. Berkley Books.

x. Ibid.

xi. Pearson, D. & Shaw, S. -1983-. Life Extension: A Practical Scientific Approach. Warner Books, Inc. P. 370.

xii. Stress researcher and author Lt. Col. -retd.- Dave Grossman explained that undercover drug agents were less likely to be killed or injured when they met with drug dealers during a meal.

xiii. Stevenson, R.K. -2014-. Backward Running. CreateSpace.

xiv. https://www.revolvy.com/topic/Bill%20%E2%80%9CBojangles%E2%80%9D%20Robinson&item_type=topic

xv. Bill Robinson. -2020, December 11-. In Wikipedia. https://en.wikipedia.org/wiki/Bill_Robinson#Shirley_Temple

xvi. Reflexology is the practice of massaging points on the feet to improve health conditions. I have been using it successfully for decades for backaches, allergies and digestive problems.

xvii. Shmerling, R. H. -2019-. The latest on glucosamine/chondroitin supplements. Harvard Health Blog. Retrieved from https://www.health.harvard.edu/blog/the-latest-on-glucosaminechondroitin-supplements-2016101710391

xviii. Mathews-Larson, J -1997- Seven Weeks to Sobriety: The Proven Program to Fight Alcoholism Through Nutrition, Ballantyne Publishing Group: New York. P. 126

xix. Rodale, J. I. & Taub, H. J. -1971-. Magnesium: The Nutrient That Could Change Your Life. Pyramid Books. Retrieved from http://www.mgwater.com/rod19.shtml
Sisk, L. -2009-. Taking Back Control. Aquarian Body Science.

xx. St. John's Wort can be purchased in health food and some drug stores. I pick mine wild at railroad tracks, parks and along some roads. It is a yellow flower easily recognized.

Discover how you can have a strong, active body at age 50 and beyond.

Based on decades of fitness and health research and interviews with high-performing active women., FIT FEMME: AFTER 50: A Busy Woman's Guide to a Strong, Attractive, Pain-Free Body will guide the reader through:

- The high energy woman's mindset. -It is not what you might think.-
- Mental reprogramming that helps push you past procrastination and whatever "they" say.
- Correcting muscle imbalances that impede your progress or cripple you with pain.
- Power nutrition to boost your endurance, strength and cognitive abilities.
- Inexpensive methods to help reduce arthritic pain
- Breathing methods that narrow your waistline.
- Detoxifying your body, mind and life.
- Achieving deep, restorative sleep.

"For years, I suffered arthritis and bursitis pain in my shoulder, back and hip. Since I joined your class, my body healed, the pain went away and I no longer needed medication. Mr. Setter, thank you so much for the freedom of working out without pain and being able to wear a size 3 dress again." Cora Lindop, Vancouver, B.C.
"There used to be a straight line from my heels to my back.
Now, I actually have a butt. Thanks Doug." -Darlene McEvoy, Grandmother, University of Manitoba

Doug Setter is an award winning author, former paratrooper, U.N. Peacekeeper, champion kick-boxer and personal trainer. He is the author of Flat Gut After 50, Reduce Your Alcohol Craving, One Less Victim and the novel Selo. Doug draws on his vast life experience to change his reader's lives. He lives in Vancouver, Canada.

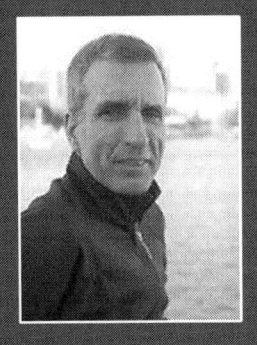

Manufactured by Amazon.ca
Bolton, ON